SKILLED VISIONS

EASA Series
Published in Association with the European Association of Social-Anthropologists (EASA)

1. LEARNING FIELDS
   Volume 1
   Educational Histories of European Social Anthropology
   Edited by Dorle Drackle, Iain R. Edgar and Thomas K. Schippers

2. LEARNING FIELDS
   Volume 2
   Current Policies and Practices in European Social Anthropology Education
   Edited by Dorle Drackle and Iain R. Edgar

3. GRAMMARS OF IDENTITY/ALTERITY
   Edited by Gerd Baumann and Andre Gingrich

4. MULTIPLE MEDICAL REALITIES
   Patients and Healers in Biomedical, Alternative and Traditional Medicine
   Edited by Helle Johannessen and Imre Lázár

5. FRACTURING RESEMBLANCES
   Identity and Mimetic Conflict in Melanesia and the West
   Simon Harrison

6. SKILLED VISIONS
   Between Apprenticeship and Standards
   Cristina Grasseni

Skilled Visions

Between Apprenticeship and Standards

Edited by

Cristina Grasseni

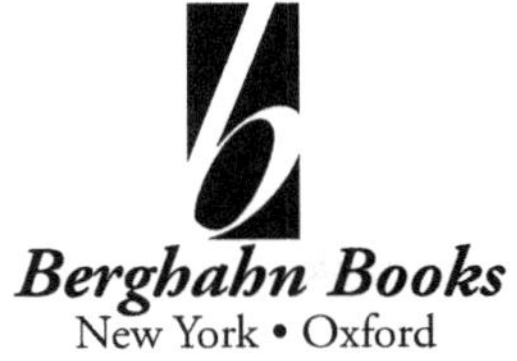

Berghahn Books
New York • Oxford

First published in 2009 by

Berghahn Books
www.berghahnbooks.com

First paperback edition published in 2010

Library of Congress Cataloging-in-Publication Data

Enduring socialism : explorations of revolution and transformation, restoration and continuation / edited by Harry G. West and Parvathi Raman. -- 1st ed.

p. cm.

Includes bibliographical references and index.

ISBN 978-1-84545-464-7 (hbk : alk. paper)

ISBN 978-1-84545-713-6 (pbk : alk. paper)

1. Post-communism. 2. Socialism. 3. Communism. I. West, Harry G. II. Raman, Parvathi.

HX44.5.E63 2008

335--dc22

2008032548

British Library Cataloguing in Publication Data

A catalogue record for this book is available from the British Library.

Printed on acid-free paper.

ISBN 978-1-84545-464-7 (hardback) -- ISBN 978-1-84545-713-6 (paperback)

Contents

List of Figures

Introduction

Skilled Visions: Between Apprenticeship and Standards

Cristina Grasseni

The object we see ...
is dependent upon who we are
and what we recognize from past experience.
(R. Arnheim, *Visual Thinking*)

Towards a Rehabilitation of Vision

Anthropologists are ready to address a yet untapped problem that is ripe for discussion: the issue of the rehabilitation of vision. The aim of this book is to propose a new concept of vision that allows us to recontextualise the critique of visualism in the wider contemporary debate on practice and the construction of knowledge. *Skilled Visions* explores the training of vision in professional, scientific and everyday settings, providing a comprehensive spectrum of case studies in relevant contexts. Local and indigenous knowledge is profiled not as a given, but in its making and in its complex relation with the hegemony of the sociotechnical network. By maintaining an ethnographic approach, the aim is to provide practical case studies that are at once accessible, critical and informative. As a whole, this work builds upon the recent literature on the anthropology of the senses: it does not consider vision as an isolated given but within its interplay with the other senses, and with the role of mutual gestuality. Moreover, it explores vision as a ductile, situated, contested and politically fraught means of situating oneself in a community of practice. By drawing together both ethnographic and sociohistorical case studies from different disciplines (especially anthropology, but also the history and sociology of science), it aims at adding further dimensions to the anthropological debate on vision.

A vast literature has concentrated on vision, and the ways in which it is being tackled by anthropologists is telling of the very same tension at the heart of the discipline, between distance and proximity.[1] On the one hand, visual media have a high profile in those processes that enforce the technological mediation of knowledge. On the other hand, vision is being recontextualised within a newly rediscovered phenomenology of the senses. Either option points towards a convergent direction. In fact, a critical focus on imaging technologies as mediators of meaning, power and knowledge often leads to an often implicit dislike of vision *tout court*, meant as synonym for the overview, the gaze, or the panoptic. The phenomenology of the senses (see Casey 1996; Jackson 1983, 1996) is often associated with a similar distancing from vision, since most arguments for a rediscovery of the body and the senses hinge on a critique of the 'visualism' of our globalised, image-driven, technified society.

Famously, Johannes Fabian's critique denounced the distancing and anachronistic bias that would be inherent in the culture of vision. Being characteristic of both Western science and the European encounters with the 'other', a certain European vision undoubtedly served as a powerful rhetoric of appropriation (see for instance Bleichmar's chapter in this book). The 'double visual fixation' of anthropological objects, 'as perceptual image and as illustration of a kind of knowledge', would also have served mainly as a distancing device that denies coevalness from the start (1983: 121). However, the recent literature in the anthropology of the senses has established that vision is cultural, and that different cultures hold radically different metaphors and hierarchy for the senses than the Western, visualist tradition (e.g. Howes 1991, 2004). Constance Classen has investigated historically and ethnographically the different symbolic investment and cultural codes of perception that societies ascribe to different senses (1993, 2005). Nadia Seremetakis (1994) has pointed out the direct link between memory, material culture and the senses. Steven Feld and Keith Basso (1996), and Paul Stoller (1989, 1997), amongst others, have focused on the sensual phenomenology of everyday practice, and the way this is linked to the construction of knowledge and the positioning of persons in their worlds.

The very realisation of the complexity and variety of sensory cultures, nevertheless, has often led to a sweeping condemnation of vision, taken *as a whole* as dominant *gaze*. The historical roots of such iconoclastic stances in literature and even photography and film are magisterially exposed by Martin Jay in his *Downcast eyes* (1993). The 'anti-ocularcentric' neologism summarises the history of ideas from Plato to Levinas, revealing a surprisingly consistent and insistent anti-visualist streak in Western intellectual history. The book is not an anti-ocularcentric manifesto, though, and the proposed alternative to ocularcentric regimes does not go beyond the proposed proliferation of diverse 'scopic regimes'. This would mean, for instance, recuperating the sense of care suggested by the etymology of 'visual' verbs both in European and non-European languages, rather than that of controlling surveillance (Jay 2002: 89).[2] Jay's analysis admittedly pertains to the *discourse* on visuality, not to the *practices* of vision. It is, instead, when we look at practice that the denunciation of gaze as per se dominating, and of vision as per se abstracting and formalising, finds an experiential check. So, while Howes (1991) and Classen (1993) rightly resist the dominant metaphors (whether visual or discursive) that treat societies as texts, the sweeping statement that anthropologists should 'resist the hegemony of the visual faculty (and the imperialist order it supports)' (Howes 1991: 19) raises some reservations. In fact, Jay testifies that in the history of art, '*optical virtuosi* with the gifts and the training to explore and extend the limits of visual experience, transcend the conventions of their visual environment and open up new worlds for our eyes' (2002: 88). This definition of *virtuoso* can be extended to those practitioners who daily go about defining and creatively extending the 'visual environments' of their practice. Cattle breeders, archaeologists, laser surgeons, even police consultants (Goodwin 1994) do each have a different world in front of their eyes, because they were each trained to see it differently, some being more gifted *virtuosi* than others.

Even though Fabian maintains a clear distinction between visualism as a cognitive style, and visual experience (if for nothing else, to warn that the former is likely to prejudice the study of the latter), his critique seems to have engendered a generalised anthropological embarrassment with the sense of vision and with visual artefacts, including a peculiar tendency to self-flagellation within visual anthropology. Such uneasiness with vision also derives from the critical analysis of the powerful discourse and the panoptic settings behind the history of imaging technologies (from the press to the media to medical settings). The success of the map and of the overview, or, as Bruno Latour would put it, of the technologies of 'inscription' and 'mediation', can hardly be explained away as mere ideology, nor can they be substituted by just 'looking at' something. (For example, the chapter by Turnbull in this book adds historical insight to the role of the map as a flexible device, both cognitive and practical). But while what Fabian objects to is in fact panopticism, as a result of a naïve reading of his critique anthropology as a discipline has often positioned itself as inherently at odds with vision, taken as a whole to stand for the chauvinistic, Western, colonial, and technified 'gaze'. This assumption has led to a lack of actual research on the processes of visual 'enskilment', that is, on the apprenticeship of *particular* skilled visions that are *specific* to *situated* practices, and on how much these can tell us about hegemony and resistance. All this *despite* the increasing interest, among the current generation of ethnographers, for the scope and reach of visual research methods (Pink et al., 2004) and for the intertwining histories of photography, film and anthropology (Grimshaw 2001; Edwards 2001) – an interest that can only benefit from the historical awareness of the many links between science and the visual arts (Galison, Jones, 1998), and from collaborative research and production across the arts and sciences (Schneider and Wright, forthcoming).

Attempts to assess vision anthropologically have so far lacked an analytical ethnographic and historical approach, preferring to stress the perceptive sensibility, personal empathy and holism that should arise from 'being there', from 'free association' or from 'sharing' a landscape with one's ethnographic subjects (Okely 1998, 2001).[3] The stress in this book is instead on the disciplined and disciplining aspects of memory and sensibility that are not spontaneous, personal and subjective but rather *embedded* in mediating devices, contexts and routines. In other words, we look here at the role of informal, mostly tacit knowledge in expert conduct, apprenticeship and professional identity, taking into consideration the role played by peer-to-peer negotiation, hierarchical relations and the management of contexts, narratives and artefacts in the social construction of skilled visions.

The accusation that visual artefacts have aided digitisation, quantification and diagrammatic representation is hard to reject. But standardisation does not apply uniquely to vision.[4] On the contrary, an investigation of visual practices in their skilled and contextual dimension may add important insights into whichever margins may be left for local negotiations by the hegemony of standards, *and* by the hierarchical order imposed in apprenticeship. This has little to do with *visualism* meant as 'a cultural, ideological bias toward vision as the noblest sense' (Fabian 1983: 106), or with the conviction, which I would keep distinct from the former, that 'to "visualise" a culture or society almost becomes synonymous for understanding it' (Fabian 1983: 106). In fact, the point of introducing the concept of skilled visions (in the plural) is precisely that of underlining how vision is not necessarily identifiable with 'detached observation', and should not be opposed by definition to 'the immediacy of fleeting sounds, ineffable odours, confused emotions, and the flow of Time passing' (108). On the contrary, *skilled visions* are embedded in multi-sensory practices, where look is coordinated with skilled movement, with rapidly changing points of view, or with other senses, such as touch. They also have a political dimension that depends on the artefacts, hierarchies and modes of exposure to local knowledges that we see described in detail in the following chapters. In other words, a simplistic reading of Fabian's critique of visualism may well still reinforce a classification of the senses whereby vision towers over the others, either as the noblest sense or as the most damning.

In a way this debate rehearses, on the one hand, the now largely 'imploded' debate on literacy (see Goody 1977; Ong 1982) and, on the other hand, on the phenomenology of space in human geography (Yi-Fu Tuan 1977; Seamon and Mugerauer 1985). Recently, an anthropological revisitation of such topics in the light of ecological psychology has led to the sketching of a new trend in ecological anthropology (see Ingold 2000). Ethno-methodological studies of science, then, have focused on detailed analyses of the various styles of vision that are effectively employed in situated practices, on their socialisation through apprenticeship and on their hegemonic potential (see for instance Goodwin and Ueno 2000; Lynch and Woolgar 1990). In visual anthropology, Anna Grimshaw (2001) has traced the many parallels and conjunctures between the history of anthropology and that of cinema, highlighting the presence of different, competing and contradictory ways of seeing, while an outspoken rehabilitation of vision as a sense of discernment in the history of art and science was outlined in Barbara Stafford's work (1996). In this book, instead of concentrating on the analysis of ready-made visual productions (whether scientific representations, artworks or documentary films) we strive to develop an anthropology *of vision* by investigating the actual processes of visual training that engender certain kinds of sociality, ideology and standards of practice. The argument proposed here is constructivist in kind: that skilled visions orient perception and structure understanding, in other words that they not only convey ideas, meaning and beliefs, but configure them. In art history and visual studies it has been argued that 'the digital imaging revolution' – for reasons that concern the technological form of mediation, transmission and representation of knowledge – 'is crucially reconfiguring how we explore and comprehend *ideas*, from urban planning to photography' (Stafford 1996: 3). Here we extend our attention for artefacts, contexts and apprenticeship to *any* instance of practices of looking.

The challenge behind this book is thus to recontextualise and possibly rephrase the debate on ocularcentrism by pursuing a new concept of *visions*, meant in the plural as local and shared practices, naturally connected to the other senses. This means taking into account the critique of panoptic vision, by opposing skilled visions, in the plural, to it. In other words, vision takes on a new meaning in a post-Fabian critical era, without avoiding the topic of vision *tout court* – as many anthropologists have done as a result of a shallow reading of such critique. To do so means situating 'skilled vision' in relation to the anthropology of practice (Chaiklin and Lave 1993; Schatzki et al. 2001) and the anthropology of the senses.

The conviction that artefacts are powerful mediators, and generators of sense, is widespread in some quarters of cultural psychology and cognitive – ecological research. Indeed, as recent literature on distributed cognition demonstrates, technological or 'cognitive' artefacts may be instrumental in mediating skill (Cole and Holland 1995; Engeström and Middleton 1996; Hutchins 1995). Recently, a vast literature has focused on a style of ethnographic research that studies the ways in which the social and material environment is organised, and how this has implications for the ways in which we understand and act in the world. However 'cognitively' oriented, these works are distinct from both the representationalist and the connectionist positions of the cognitive sciences.[5] Their main tenet is the idea that cognition is the result of the interaction of actors and objects, which arrange specific practices in local contexts. So human congnition, unlike that of computers, is not a question of implementing algorythms but is *embodied*, relational and interactive, hence social (Varela et al. 1991; Whitehouse 2001). From the stepping stones represented by the works of Michael Cole, Edwin Hutchins, Jean Lave and Lucy Suchman, anthropological research on cognition has developed as a study of *situated action*. Though coming from different backgrounds (in anthropology, linguistics and psychology) these works share a set of main tenets regarding social action. Firstly, they consider *mediated action* as crucial to practice (as in the different traditions of Dewey's pragmatism, G.H. Mead's interactionism, Bateson's ecology of mind, and above all the cultural-historical Russian school of Lev Vygotsky, Alexei Leont'ev and Alexander Luria[6]). Secondly, they focus on environmental systems, including both material and relational structures, underlying the recursive, co-constitutive and co-evolving dynamics that organise them. As a species capable of mediated action, humankind banks on the socially guided appropriation of environmental resources that are oriented to practice by the previous generations. Environmental systems are hence external sources of memory and knowledge which sediment through generations and which are accessed through socialisation (Cole 1997). Thirdly, humans find themselves continuously involved in *performances* and *routines* that allow them to share common fields of action. Culture therefore takes the shape of a set of resources that can be employed creatively in different ways by the social actors: cultural action is the *situated improvisation* that exploits such resources in different circumstances, rather than an interpretative frame or a fixed repertoire. In turn, contexts are mutually constituted by people's actions rather than fixed scenarios for them.

Capitalising on this literature, but privileging its ethnographic rather than its psychological potential, means applying it to a methodological enquiry about the ethnographic relevance of what we could term 'practices of locality'.[7] The interdisciplinary work that has been developed in this book adds to this literature, and distinguishes itself from it, for a closer ethnographic look at *context* in its wider sense. This means looking into issues such as: where artefacts come from (see chapters by Grasseni, Bleichmar, Turnbull); how they are inserted into roles, narratives and prefigured hierarchies of power, contributing to their preservation (Saunders, Roepstorff, Cohn), and what margins – if any – are left to innovation, creativity and disruption (Ronzon, Gunn, Willerslev). The invitation made to the authors was to explore the ways in which vision can be shared across a community as *an enskilled sense*, to highlight the processes of apprenticeship that refine vision as a skilled *capacity*, and to focus on the institutional audiences and the contexts of labour that have historically engaged vision as a specific *form of practice*.

In order to introduce and in some ways limit the possible interpretations of the notion of 'skilled visions', it may be useful to stress what is *not* the object of this agenda. 'Skilled vision' is not a metaphor for *knowledge tout court*, nor a synonym for *observation*, nor an invitation to exercise critical analysis of particular visual *representations*. The aim is to show how there is no neutral and detached gaze, but rather that there are different practices of *looking*, and that learning some 'good looking' (Stafford 1996) is inevitably part (and a necessary precondition) of insight into such practices. Far from being exercises in neutral observation, then, skilled visions can be analysed in terms of practical routines, social and ideological *belonging* as well as of aesthetic *longing*. Moreover, skilled visions are not necessarily related to image-making processes, so that studying skilled visions does not necessarily mean conducting a critical reading of visual artefacts. To sum up, skilled visions are the result of concrete processes of education of attention, within situated practices and ecologies of culture that are at the same time 'vulnerable, unruly, and evanescent as well as contested, collective, and distributed', as Simon Schaffer so aptly pinpointed.[8] I wish to dwell for a few paragraphs on each of these characteristics.

Collective and distributed. The role of communities of practice (Lave and Wenger 1991; Wenger 1998), and of their shared ways of seeing, can be shown to be far from residual in producing collective and active belonging to aesthetic ideals, moral order and standards of accomplishment. Skilled visions often rely on collaborative expertise and on a distribution of cognitive artefacts that are made available and relevant in the landscape of one's practice – or *taskscape* (Ingold 1993). They often entail a capacity to discriminate: one may well isolate one trait from the flux of one's sensorial experience, if this is more relevant or fundamental to one's taskscape. Skilled visions cannot be associated solely with the use of specific visual media, or with image-making processes (video, film, digital photography, paper, wood, or imaging software). Nor, once acquired, are they bound to the use of a certain visual environment or medium.[9]

Vulnerable and unruly. Whilst forms of image-making may be the principal engagement of such skilled practices, one should also underline the vaster scopes of visual practices. Some are aimed at making one *see as*, that is to acquire certain patterns of expert scrutiny, which one applies to diverse configurations of objects. Applying such patterns is also a question of making one's expertise *visible to others*. Thirdly, skilled visions may also involve the ability to *see through* grids, ideal types and standard artefacts as much as that of 'seeing as'. In other words, different schoolings may allow differently trained people to derive different, or conflicting information, from the same visual artefact. Conversely, the ability to trace, view and make use of different artefacts coherently marks the social and cognitive – often ideologically biased – cohesion of a community of practice.

Contested and evanescent. Skilled visions are in fact ambivalent and omnipresent. The local construction of skilled knowledge, through the training of expert eyes, hands, discourses and sensibilities, actually contributes to the establishment and maintenance of hegemonic, often global, standards of practice through which we perceive, order and manage the world. The highly selective, prescriptive and binding routines of professional locales becomes transparent, like a pair of glasses to look through, to its practitioners through training, and precisely for this reason it can be ideological and hegemonic. Hence the situated practices of laboratories, hospitals and offices constitute key steps towards the assimilation, and sometimes the negotiation, of global hierarchies of value (Herzfeld 2004). Is there any space left for resistance and creativity? This is one of the questions this book wishes to ask. In architectural practices, medical laboratories, marginal rural areas and urban wastelands, peasants, medical apprentices, artists and performers strive to manage the required compromise between distance and proximity, between locality and globality, between individual skill and political sociality. Often these very strategies reinstate the marginality and subalternity of their protagonists.

Situating Skilled Visions: Between Apprenticeship and Standards

I stated above that in order to move beyond the critique of ocularcentrism we need to re-contextualise the idea of vision itself within the dialectics between locality and the network, as part of a social construction of meaning. Within this dialectic, as Herzfeld notices in his Epilogue to this book, skilled vision is placed in a pivotal position: between apprenticeship and standards. As I pointed out in the previous section, ethnographies of scientific, professional and organisational contexts have argued that human activity is mediated by artefacts (Norman 1988; Suchman 1987) which often have a standardising function. In particular, the visual and situated component of human interaction and communication has been demonstrated (Goodwin 1994, 1998). On the other hand, from phenomenological and ecological quarters it has been stressed how educating attention involves multi-sensory experience and personal apprenticeship (Ingold 2000). Is this a contradiction? Is it a contradiction that both apprenticeship *and* standard artefacts mediate the situated, tacit, skilful knowledge of individuals in communities of practice (Lave and Wenger 1991)? The thesis of this book is that situated practices do not per se contradict the 'metropolitan' and 'metrological' nature of technological mediation that is achieved through the dissemination of mobile inscriptions (Latour 1991). On the contrary, they make it work and often guarantee its ideological success by disseminating it in local contexts.

The following chapters show how vision is a powerful carrier of knowledge, sociality and identity: a successful go-between from the grounded, situated body to the global hierarchies of sociotechnical networks. Vision is analysed here not as a metaphor for something else, but as an actual process that characterises everyday life in different communities of practice. Instead of simply accepting that vision is 'cultural', hence rehearsing the argument of cultural relativism but leaving the actual problem of mapping 'culture' untapped, these case studies address the difference it makes to personal identities, social relations and professional ideologies to be trained in one way of seeing rather than another. The ambition of this research agenda is to address squarely, both in theoretical terms and through reference to a wide spectrum of ethnographic and historical settings, the issue of how we *see*. This is a missing link in contemporary theory on global–local dynamics: we cannot understand how people function unless we take into consideration how they have learnt to see the world in many different, relevant and conflicting ways.

The case studies presented here stress the role of *context* (both material and social), of social *relationships* (both mimetic and conflictual) and of the processes of *apprenticeship* in putting a certain vision firmly in place within a community of practice. Apprenticeship and schooling are part of a sociotechnical network, where audience, authority and artefacts play an important part. The aim, though, is not only *to acknowledge the existence* of social contexts for specific practices of seeing (professional, artistic, scientific), but *to dwell on the actual processes* through which people are trained into communities of practice by learning to relate to certain tools, narratives and categories. The agenda is hence to analyse concrete *processes* of enskilment, the role of *artefacts* in an ecology of attention, and *social historical and institutional paths* of engagement in practices. By focusing on apprenticeship, such analyses uncover the process of 'erasure of the muddling' (Herzfeld, p. 213) that is characteristic of institutional practices, while contributing ethnographic insight into modern places and high-tech environments. The scientists, medics and professionals portrayed here are shown to be 'feeling their way' around, while they are being taught exactly where and how to look for 'data'. In the ecology of everyday practice, both in professional and in marginal contexts, this highlights the ways in which ideology, beliefs, ethics and aesthetics become incorporated, hence transparent and pervasive at once.

Considering vision as a form of practice is hence a deliberate theoretical move, which allows us to supersede the current debate on visualism in favour of a more encompassing analysis, regarding the roles of *local contexts* and *community* in constituting knowledge. Here too there are contrasting interpretations. Locality and contingency in the constitution of knowledge can be simply understood as material and idiosyncratic resistances to the processes of inscription and encoding. Thanks to the powerful tools of visualisation and inscription, such resistances can be overcome so that translation, technological mediation and eventually the transportability and visibility of knowledge can be achieved. But the anthropological perception of locality as a nexus of shared relations and of practice-generating knowledge is oppositional to this perception of vision as universal translator and mediator. Consequently, recent ethnographic approaches stressing the local and relational character of knowledge-making have often been associated with anti-visualist stances. How can a revisitation of skill help to overcome such opposition? As was indicated by the theme chosen for the 2004 EASA biennial meeting, 'rethinking distance and proximity' is a fresh challenge for anthropology, as well as for the humanities and social sciences. The need to study skill comes from the fact that, while technological mediation ensures the global dissemination of standards, professional apprenticeship still constructs knowledge *locally* by training expert practitioners. Hence, rethinking the role of proximity *vis-à-vis* the standardisation of knowledge means reconsidering the many forms and roles of tacit knowledge (Polany 1958), *and* situating them in contemporary global networks of commodities and hierarchies of roles.

'Skill' is a core concept through which technology, history, social relations and political economy converge, complexifying the perception of globalisation as a predetermined discourse that implies the demise of so-called traditional skills by the hand of modern technology. In fact, there is no fixed algebra of skill and machine by which an increase of technology means a decrease in skill (see for instance Collins 1997 on medical skill in high-tech surgery). Once acquired, skill is an essential aspect, an element of practice, a taste and a meaning-making attitude that is developed and applied throughout everyday life, thus amounting to a sense of identification or emplacement (Mollona 2002). Conversely, it is the very substance of ideology in that it perpetuates self-justifying criteria of propriety and correctness that are internal to communities of practice and their hierarchies. Skill may be a way of embedding practical relations between human beings and their everyday environment (see Gray 1999). As I have argued elsewhere (Grasseni 2004 a and b), the 'correct' appreciation of beauty and grace, the sense of accomplishment and the corresponding social appreciation of skill go hand in hand: such moral order will underlie not only professional performances, but also gossip, competition, reputation, dominance etc.

One of the aims of the book is to explore vision in terms of 'enskilment', meant in this broader sense (for a narrower definition cf. Ingold 1993: 221), within an ecology of practice. One grants that the enskilment of vision goes along with the enskilment of the other senses, and in particular of bodily movement and dexterity, as part of a progressive process of joining a particular 'community of practice' – a process that Jean Lave calls 'legitimate peripheral participation'. Lave and Wenger (1991) coined this phrase to indicate the critical moment of socialisation of new actors, through apprenticeship, in specific 'communities of practice', and a fundamental mechanism of situated learning. These authors underline the unity of cognitive and operative aspects on the one side and, on the other, the socialising and relational dynamics of to-be experts. From an anthropological point of view, the concept of 'community of practice' offers a pragmatic scope for observing cognition and skill at work and in their making; it provides a social context within which locating apprenticeship as a process of 'education of attention' (Ingold 2000) that shapes specific skills of relation, cognition and perception. Firstly mimetic processes are often the socioemotional motor for the process of apprenticeship. They are, more often than not, highly conflictual (see Dumouchel and Dupuy 1982). Secondly, enskilling does not necessarily mean learning without rules, just as training vision does not exclude verbalisation. Thirdly, the capacities developed in these systems are exportable to other contexts and systems of activity. Communities of practice in fact provide a social and cognitive horizon that justifies and reproduces specific contexts of perception action, and within which resonance or attunement, rather than actual communication, support understanding (Wikan 1993).

To sum up, skilled practices literally shape the way we look at the world. Participating in a richly textured environment, full of objects, images and body patterns, structures and guides our perception tacitly and implicitly. In the naturally and culturally constructed environments we thus inhabit, identity and cultures are rooted and reproduce themselves. 'Sharing a worldview' may thus mean learning to inhabit ecologies of vision, taken as 'the public organisation of visual practice within the worklife of a profession' (Goodwin 2000: 164). The notions of *taskscape* (Ingold) and *worldview* thus converge on the issue of practical understanding, achieved locally through material and social learning experiences. A sense of propriety, of aesthetic accomplishment and of moral order is developed and transmitted in communities of practice. I refer here to the identity-making processes through which, by encountering, perceiving and investing the objects and spaces of everyday activity with meaning, people form attachments and a sense of themselves. Skilled visions, once acquired, are not so much codes, or tools for actively manipulating messages, as much as backgrounds and scenarios that make those messages meaningful. The fact that practice can engender *understanding* as a sediment of experience and skill raises issues of commensurability (Hollis and Lukes 1982) that I shall not deal with in depth here (see Grasseni, forthcoming). It suffices to say, for the purposes of this book, that acquiring specific skills may help the ethnographer to access worldviews and to document how ways of knowing are embedded in social practice. Ecologies of practice orient not only strategies for developing ethnographic participation and field relations, but also a theoretical search for the ways and tools through which everyday activities are organised (spatially, socially, cognitively).

The Structure of the Book

As should be clear by now, the thesis of this book is that to exercise skilled vision means to belong socially in communities and networks that share aesthetic sensibilities, principles of good practice, rituals of participation, processes of apprenticeship, ideological stances and political interests. Each chapter focuses on the making of different skilled visions, meant as situated and embodied practices that can provide anthropological insight into identity, conflict and ideology. The book opens by giving a varied insight into what 'ecology of practice' may mean in relation to skilled visions, by stressing the relevance of local aesthetics both in traditional, rural spaces and in urban, less conventional settings (Part I). Part II positions the role of gestuality and of embodied practice in relation to the concept of *design*, seen at work in art, architecture and neuro-imaging. Part III revisits, in the light of the notions of skilled visions, the social, political and technical relevance of visual training in scientific and medical practice. The chapters articulate an interdisciplinary approach, underlining different historical, sociological and ethnographic dimensions of skilled visions. The fields of skilled practice investigated span architecture, art, ethnographic research, urban planning, neuroscience, medical training, transvestitism, hunting and breeding, including examples of visual training in both high- and low-tech environments, and relevant historical and epistemological perspectives. Each section proposes *complementary and comparative views* from interdisciplinary research (mostly anthropological, but also sociohistorical and science-historical) on different areas of practice. *Showing by contrast* is both a strategy for apprenticeship and the style of these case studies. For example, brain imaging is compared to navigating skills; wood-sculpting to C.A.D. (computer-aided design) drawing; the Linnaean botanical drawings used in colonial botany are compared against pictorial production in the colonies; the skills of medieval masonry with the ones of managing the London underground traffic. The apprenticeship of beauty is analysed in such apparently disparate contexts as animal husbandry and transvestite performance. This collection of historical and ethnographic cases shows the different ways in which training vision means shaping professional identities, negotiating personal ability and conveying hegemonic values. From this focused viewpoint, one appreciates the social dynamics at work in professional apprenticeship and training, covering a wide historical, science-historical and ethnographic scope, showing how a global network of standards influences local definitions of knowledge, beauty and good practice. Particular attention is given to the sensory, discursive and cognitive strategies of marginality and resistance both in professional and everyday practice.

The first section of the book explores different skilled visions in the ecologies of everyday practice at the margins of the global hierarchy of value. Rane Willerslev argues head-on for a pro-visual stance: 'surely there must be more to vision than the indefinite number of practical contexts in which it is employed?' He draws on phenomenologist Merleau-Ponty to argue in favour of the distancing element that vision, unlike the other senses, introduces into our sensuous relation to the world: 'in vision, distance and proximity are not mutually exclusive, but rather imply one another' (p. 25). The case of the perspectivism of Yukaghir hunters is brought to illustrate the case. Hunters and elks have to undergo a process of mimetic transformation that results in increased affinity between them, a process that entails all the senses and is aimed at seducing the prey into self-surrender. But hunters must be careful not to get too close to the prey lest they 'go native' and fail the hunt. Moreover, Willerslev argues that the distance afforded by sight 'allows the subject not only to be aware of the visible world but also to be in a fundamental way aware of his own visibility, his own activity of seeing' (p. 30). It is this self-awareness that negotiates the liminality between distance and proximity – a compromise which ultimately safeguards the self from mimetic dissolution. The argument is in keeping with the project of the rehabilitation of vision, meant as a skilled sense that both allows and requires discernment, disciplining and awareness. It applies not only to the Yukaghir hunter but to the anthropologist herself: rather than giving in to the seduction of sensuous immersion, she should practise the liminality of differentiation.

In the second chapter, I combine historical and ethnographic perspectives in order to follow up the traces of apparently *transparent* artefacts such as plastic toy cows, sketching out the historical development of a 'breeding aesthetics' that is currently associated with intensive dairy farming. The apprenticeship into the skilled vision of breed selection eventually attunes one to an intimate appreciation of what are deemed ideologically as 'good looking' animals – even though these criteria eventually depend on the complex history of animal husbandry and breed selection, and on the economic imperatives of competitive intensive production. Amongst breeders' children, toys play a functional role in the social mimicry of adult expertise. The creative, performative and narrative use of such toys parallels the cognitive and social role played by scale models of 'ideal cows' in the settings of their parents' professional life. Scale models serve, in fact, as trophies and prizes of cattle fairs and are exhibited in both domestic and professional contexts, thus serving both an educational purpose and one of social acknowledgement.

Francesco Ronzon elaborates on irony, cognition and visual skill from the margins of acceptable theatrical performance, following a group of drag queens acting on stage in the gay clubs of Verona (Italy). Ronzon explores Madame Sisi's aesthetic sensibility and breaks down 'camp as a way of seeing' into the artefacts, icons and verbal exchanges that ecologically support, cognitively mediate and socially acknowledge drag-queen interpretations and performances of 'propriety' and of 'beauty'. Here, 'skilled vision' is the result of verbal, optical and aesthetic training carried out as resistance in the face of historical discrimination and marginalisation. The author has to 'pick up' the relevant cues and debates in an environment where commonsensical definitions of beauty and grace break down, and an alternative tradition of 'ecology of mind' is upheld.

The second section of the book maintains a combination of both historical and ethnographic focus, positioning different gestures of design in the practices of art, architecture and brain imaging. Simon Cohn compares two very different settings in which medical skill is, in the perception of its practitioners, akin to drawing: scalpel surgery and neural imaging. Both show in non-obvious ways how medicine can be perceived as both an art and a science. His analysis challenges 'a romantic notion of skill as simply being some indefinite, intuitive acquisition gained in some inexplicable way from embodied, repeated action or "raw talent", in opposition to intentional, directed, judicious learning' (p. 92). The case links up with Saunders's (ch. 9) in its focus on technological innovation, which threatens the traditional basis of practice through automatisation, digitalisation and simulation, i.e. through the introduction of powerful imaging mediators between the eye and the hand of the surgeon and its object – the body. Both in traditional and in neuro-imaging settings, though, seeing depends on the doctor's capacity to allow the body to reveal itself – a capacity that may require 'playing around' in a way that experts are more comfortable with than novices. Hence 'seeing is not a single moment of apprehension, but involves an on-going combination of recognising, acknowledging and acting upon' (p. 94). Cohn dwells on the hidden narrative, dialogical and conversational dynamics through which an 'expert community' 'orients itself towards certain images as being legitimate and meaningful'. The 'interpretive basis of medicine' is hence firmly at the core of expertise even when 'seeing' cannot be confused with naïve realism but is self-consciously the result of technological simulation.

Wendy Gunn highlights different knowledge places in relation to her own pattern of learning, considering the different meaning of *drawing* in architectural and art practices. Her personal engagement in comparative participant observation stems from the conviction that 'some forms of knowledge afforded within creative practice resist commodification and institutionalisation' (p. 109). The kind of 'skilled vision' she tries to mimic, following the Welsh artist David Nash, the Norwegian architect Knut-Eirik Dahl and students of Dundee Academy of Fine Art, is opposed to viewing from a distance. The ways in which she chooses to *observe* captures both the fluidity of sculpting gestures and the reflexivity of mimicry, the poetics of creativity and the narrativity of resistance. All this is part of a more encompassing project that aims at problematising the idea of *learning* – specifically of forms of knowledge that cannot be written down – a project that has *skill* at its core, meant as 'the very ground of knowledge, not merely its application'.

David Turnbull's chapter expands on the idea of 'performing design', taking the London Underground and Chartres Cathedral as two examples of it. Turnbull contrasts 'representationalism' and 'performativity', through a sociohistorical analysis of how the London Underground map was designed, accepted as 'traditional', and of how it informs our perception of urban space to this very day. Performativity locates 'seeing not just in forms and technologies of visualisation and representation, but in embodied performances and practices, situated, and distributed in time and place' (p. 126). In the case of Chartres Cathedral, then, what has been hailed as the epitome of a harmonious unity, or the result of architectural coherence, is revealed as 'an ad hoc mess' (p. 134). The idea of an overall design is superseded, in the analysis of historian of architecture John James, by the succession of different masons and by the role of templates. These were a key tool for communication and knowledge transmission within the 'scopic regime of the medieval world', which privileged 'skilled visual practice based in location' (p. 137).

The third section of the book is devoted to the social schooling of the eye in scientific and medical settings. Barry Saunders introduces us to the hierarchical and theatrical rites of learning radiology, focusing on reading CT scans as an example of the process of interpreting medical images. He renders a varied and diverse spectrum of the many aspects of apprenticeship – from autodidactic memorisation to exemplary demonstrations to novice performance, grounding it ethnographically in the pedagogical settings, performative roles and heuristic devices of a narrative of 'intrigue'. Here as elsewhere, visual apprenticeship goes hand in hand with other forms of dexterity, while the ambiguity of seeing leaves ample space for developing what is perceived as an 'interpretive craft' that demands and engenders aesthetic engagement, acumen and emulation – nothing to share with a mechanical 'pattern recognition'. Saunders's analysis of the disappearance of the mechanical viewbox adds an important dimension of transition and historical contingency that belongs to all processes of apprenticeship and enskilment, highlighting the tight links between communal learning, social rituality and the physical organisation of learning environments.

Daniela Bleichmar's science-historical chapter deepens the historical dimension of skilled vision with an analysis of the visual culture of botanical illustrations in the colonial science of the eighteenth century. She shows how naturalists were trained to be expert observers, and how these skills were deployed and challenged in the field. Their ideals of observation and manipulation still raise problems for the current anthropological debate on visualism. In particular, Bleichmar discusses how 'the notion of sight went beyond the physiological act of seeing to involve rather *insight*' (p. 168) – a distinction that the paradox of the *blind naturalist* brings to the fore. Complex training and expert manipulation of reference texts demonstrates once again how 'seeing was neither simple nor immediate, but a sophisticated technique that identified practitioners as belonging or not to a community of observers' (p. 175), not only according to a set of standards and practices but also to a series of attributes that became characteristic of the very persona of the naturalist.

Andreas Roepstorff raises the issue of how understanding images plays a role in the construction of skilled vision within a scientific community. Neuro-imaging is analysed as a social process involving an 'imagined community of peers', while the education of attention is once again confirmed as 'a key process in establishing the borders of the scientific community' (p. 191). Through comparison with navigational skills and through discourse analysis, Roepstorff shows how the construction and interpretation of brain images 'becomes embedded in a narrative' which is akin to 'a navigation in brainscape' (p. 198). In other words, 'images are arguments' within which, as in navigation, 'certain features stand out as facts (p. 201) during social interaction. Facts are, in Ludwig Fleck's terms, 'signs of resistance to a thought collective' (p. 202) that become 'solidified through other narratives' (p. 204).

To conclude and summarise, the aim of this collection is to develop a framework and to investigate methodologies apt to contribute to interdisciplinary discussion, focusing on the collective and distributed nature of vision and skill, on the transactions that bring about 'skilled vision', and on the mutual dynamics of (visual) recognition and (social) reciprocity. While not disputing the penetrative and dominant character that certain skilled visions may exercise in various examples of skilled practice, the invitation is to take into account the 'vulnerability, unruliness, evanescence' of its objects and the 'contested, collective and distributed' character of its practice. *Vision*, both as a theoretically dense metaphor (as worldview), and as part of a phenomenology of the senses (as vision*s*), is relevant to anthropological practice, and is not necessarily *visualist*. The ambition of this project is to establish ethnography as a methodological asset for practice theory; to start exploring the processes of apprenticeship that create identities in professional, educational and performative contexts; to suggest which forms of participant observation are needed to highlight them.

Acknowledgements

Interdisciplinary discussions around 'Skilled Visions' and situated knowledge were initiated at a preparatory seminar, 'Practices of Locality', held in 2000 at the University of Milan Bicocca with Paola Filippucci, thanks to a post-doctorate bursary on the epistemology of visual anthropology. In 2004 I organised a thematic session at the Vienna EASA Biennial Meeting and coorganised, with Mike Bravo and Andreas Roepstorff, the symposium *Skilled Visions. Educating Attention in the Field*, hosted by C.R.A.S.S.H. (Centre for Research in the Arts, Social Sciences and Humanities) at Cambridge University. The chapters in this book represent a selection of papers given at the EASA panel with invited contributions from some of the participants of the Milan and Cambridge workshops. My warmest thanks go to all those who participated in the various stages of discussion and elaboration of the notion of skilled vision. In particular, Simon Schaffer's role as a discussant at the Cambridge symposium was paramount in clarifying some of the most challenging aspects of this concept, while Michael Herzfeld acted as discussant at the Vienna meeting and engaged consistently and generously with the editorial project that ensued. The Centre for Research in the Anthropology and Epistemology of Complexity (CE.R.CO.) at the University of Bergamo (Italy) provided the ideal institutional basis for developing this project and hosted its follow-up symposium in June 2006.

Notes

1 See the key theme chosen for the EASA Biennial Meeting at Vienna in 2004: *Face to Face. Connecting Distance and Proximity.*

2 While Jay underlines the sense of care contained in the French *le regarde*, van Enk and de Vries make a similar observation of the Korowai language (1997: 42, quoted in Matera 2002: 11).

3 See also Okely's paper, 'Fieldwork as Free Association and Free Passage', at the 2004 EASA Biennial Meeting.

4 The standardisation of taste is one emerging issue in the global commodity market. Expert tasters can be trained to pin down cheese or coffee taste to a numeric value in a range of variables, and then to transcribe them into forms and diagrams (Grasseni, in preparation).

5 While the former identify cognition with the manipulation of symbols in a regulated algorithm that generates representations of the world, the latter refers to the model of parallel distributed processing of the neural networks.

6 This psychological school ascribed a central role to the historical and social processes of development, and to the *cultural artefacts* (symbols, objects and representation) that mediate human behaviour in various systems of activity.

7 As in the 'Practices of Locality' seminar held in 2000 at the University of Milan-Bicocca where, I first raised the issue of 'skilled vision' in my work on cattle breeders and the apprenticeship of ideals of good form, or animal beauty (Grasseni 2004a).

8 Simon Schaffer, *Skilled Visions Symposium*, round table discussion, Cambridge, 14th May, 2004.

9 For instance, the skilled vision of a breed expert – acquired through personal frequentation of cattle fairs and sheds – remains highly attuned even when applied to a VHS recording of a cattle fair that she may watch on television. Likewise, the same skilled vision is developed by her children through playing and manipulating model toys (see Chapter 2).

References

Arnheim, R. 1969. *Visual Thinking*. Berkeley: University of California Press.

Casey, E.S. 1996. 'How to Get from Space to Place in a Fairly Short Stretch of Time', in *Senses of Place*, eds. S. Feld and K. Basso, Seattle: School of American Research Press, 13–52.

Chaiklin, S. and J. Lave, eds. 1993. *Understanding Practice: Perspectives on Activity and Context*. Cambridge: Cambridge University Press.

Classen, C. 1993. *Worlds of Sense*. London: Routledge.

—— ed. 2005. *The Book of Touch*. Oxford: Berg.

Cole, M. 1997. *Culture and Cognitive Science*. San Diego: Laboratory of Comparative Human Cognition, on line at: http://lchc.ucsd.edu/People/Localz/MCole/santabar.html

Cole, M. and D. Holland, 1995. 'Between Discourse and Schema: Reformulating a Cultural-Historical Approach to Culture and Mind', *Anthropology and Education Quarterly* 26: 475–90.

Collins, H.M. 1997. 'Ways of Going On: an Analysis of Skill Applied to Medical Practice', *Science, Technology and Human Values* 22: 267–84.

Dumouchel P. and J.P. Dupuy, 1982. *L'auto-organisation: De la physique au politique*. Paris: Seuil.

Edwards, E. 2001. *Raw Histories: Photographs, Anthropology and Museums.* Oxford: Berg.
Engeström, Y. and D. Middleton, eds. 1998. *Cognition and Communication at Work.* Cambridge: Cambridge University Press.
Fabian, J. 1983. *Time and the Other: How Anthropology Makes its Object.* New York: Columbia University Press.
Feld, S. and K. Basso, eds. 1996. *Senses of Place.* Seattle: School of American Research Press.
Galison, P. and C. Jones, eds. 1998. *Producing Art, Picturing Science.* London: Routledge.
Goodwin, C. 1994. 'Professional Vision', *American Anthropologist* 96 (3): 606–33.
——2000. 'Practices of Seeing: Visual Analysis: an Ethnomethodological Approach', in *Handbook of Visual Analysis*, eds. T. van Leeuwen and C. Jewitt. London: Sage Publications, 157–82.
Goodwin, C. and M.H. Goodwin, 1998. 'Formulating Planes: Seeing as a Situated Activity', in *Cognition and Communication at Work*, eds. D. Middleton, and Y. Engeström. Cambridge: Cambridge University Press.
Goodwin, C. and N. Ueno, eds. 2000. *Vision and Inscription in Practice.* Special issue of *Mind, Culture and Activity* 7 (1–2).
Goody, J. 1977. *The Domestication of the Savage Mind.* Cambridge: Cambridge University Press.
Grasseni, C. 2004a. 'Skilled Vision. An Apprenticeship in Breeding Aesthetics', *Social Anthropology* 12 (1): 1–15.
——2004b. 'Skilled Landscapes: Mapping Practices of Locality', *Environment and Planning D: Society and Space* 22: 699–717.
——in preparation. *Reinventing food: Organic Views: Viewing Cultures of Taste at the Feet of the Alps.*
——Forthcoming 2007. 'Communities of Practice and Forms of Life: Towards a Rehabilitation of Anthropological Vision?', in *Ways of Knowing*, ed. Mark Harris. Oxford: Berghahn Books.
Gray, J. 1999. 'Open Spaces, Dwelling Places: Being at Home on Hill Farms in the Scottish Borders', *American Ethnologist* 26 (2): 440–60.
Grimshaw, A. 2001. *The Ethnographer's Eye: Ways of Seeing in Anthropology.* Cambridge: Cambridge University Press.
Herzfeld, M. 2004. *The Body Impolitic: Artisans and Artifice in the Global Hierarchy of Value.* Chicago: Chicago University Press.
Hollis, M. and S. Lukes, eds. 1982. *Rationality and Relativism.* Oxford: Basil Blackwell.
Howes, D. 1991. *The Varieties of Sensory Experience: A Sourcebook in the Anthropology of the Senses.* Toronto: University of Toronto Press.
——ed 2004. *Empire of the Senses: The Sensual Culture Reader.* Oxford: Berg.
Hutchins, E. 1995. *Cognition in the Wild.* Cambridge, Mass.: MIT Press.
Ingold, T. 1993. 'The Art of Translation in a Continuous World', in *Beyond Boundaries: Understanding, Translation and Anthropological Discourse*, ed. G. Pálsson. London: Berg, 210–30.
——2000. *The Perception of the Environment: Essays in Livelihood, Dwelling and Skill.* London: Routledge.
Jackson, M. 1983. 'Knowledge of the Body', *Man* 18: 327–45.
——1996. 'Introduction: Phenomenology, Radical Empiricism, and Anthropological Critique', in *Things As They Are. New Directions in Phenomenological Anthropology*, ed. M. Jackson. Bloomington: Indiana University Press.

Jay, M. 1993. *Downcast Eyes. The Denigration of Vision in Twentieth-Century French Thought*. Berkeley: University of California Press.

——2002 'That Visual Turn. The Advent of Visual Culture', *Journal of Visual Culture* 1 (1): 87–92.

Latour, B. 1991. *Nous n'avons jamais été modernes*. Paris: Editions La Découverte.

Lave, J. and E. Wenger, 1991. *Situated Learning: Legitimate Peripheral Participation*. Cambridge: Cambridge University Press.

Lynch, M. and S. Woolgar, eds. 1990. *Representation in Scientific Practice*. Cambridge, Mass.: MIT Press.

Matera, V. 2002. 'Antropologia dei sensi. Osservazioni introduttive', *Ricerca Folklorica* 45: 7–28.

Mollona, M. 2002. 'Ceux du≪chaud≫ ceux du ≪froid≫. Fabriquer des outils à Sheffield', *Terrain* 39: 93–108.

Norman, D. 1988. *The Psychology of Everyday Things*. New York: Basic Books.

Okely, J. 1998. 'Picturing and Placing Constable Country', in *Siting Culture*, eds. K. Fog Olwig and K. Hastrup. London: Routledge.

——2001. 'Visualism and Landscape: Looking and Seeing in Normandy', *Ethnos* 66: 99–120.

Ong, W. 1982. *Orality and Literacy: The Technologizing of the Word*. London: Methuen.

Pink, S., A. Afonso and L. Kurti, eds. 2004. *Working Images*: Visual Research and Representation in Ethnography. London: Routledge.

Polanyi, M. 1958. *Personal Knowledge: Towards a Post-critical Philosophy*. Chicago: University of Chicago Press.

Schatzki, T., K. Knorr Cetina and E. von Savigny, eds. 2001. *The Practice Turn in Contemporary Theory*. London: Routledge.

Schneider, A. and C. Wright, eds. Forthcoming. *Fieldworks: Dialogues between Art and Anthropology*. London: Berg.

Seamon, D. and R. Mugerauer, eds. 1985. *Dwelling, Place and Environment. Towards a Phenomenology of Person and World*. New York: Columbia University Press.

Seremetakis, N. 1994. *The Senses Still: Perception and Memory as Material Culture in Modernity*. Chicago: University of Chicago Press.

Stafford, B.M. 1996. *Good Looking: Essays on the Virtue of Images*. Cambridge, Mass.: MIT Press.

Stoller, P. 1989. *The Taste of Ethnographic Things: The Senses in Anthropology*. Philadelphia: University of Pennsylvania Press.

——1997. *Sensuous Scholarship*. Philadelphia: University of Pennsylvania Press.

Suchman, L. 1987. *Plans and Situated Action: The Problem of Human–Machine Communication*. Cambridge: Cambridge University Press.

Varela, F., E. Thompson and E. Rosch, 1991. *The Embodied Mind: Cognitive Science and Human Experience*. Cambridge, Mass.: MIT Press.

Wenger, E. 1998. *Communities of Practice: Learning, Meaning and Identity*. Cambridge: Cambridge University Press.

Whitehouse, H., ed. 2001. *The Debated Mind: Evolutionary Psychology versus Ethnography*. Oxford: Berg.

Wikan, U. 1993. 'Beyond the Words. The Power of Resonance', in *Beyond Boundaries: Understanding, Translation and Anthropological Discourse*, ed. G. Pálsson. London: Berg, 184–209.

Yi-Fu Tuan. 1977. *Space and Place: The Perspective of Experience*. Minneapolis: University of Minnesota Press.

Part I

Skilled Visions and the Ecology of Practice

Chapter 1

'To have the world at a distance': Reconsidering the Significance of Vision for Social Anthropology

Rane Willerslev

And yet, although at one with the world, the painter is also apart from it, which is the paradoxical, enigmatic 'madness' of vision: 'Painting awakens and carries to its highest pitch a delirium which is vision itself, for to see is *to have at a distance.*'
Merleau-Ponty (1964) quoted in Jay (1994: 314–15)

Introduction

The recent conviction that anthropology, as a European project, is marked by an ocularcentric paradigm has caused much anxiety about vision within the discipline. Thus, during the 1980s, Fabian (1983: 106) famously launched a criticism against the dominance of the visual in social anthropology, arguing that the discipline's 'cultural, ideological bias towards vision as the noblest sense' leads the fieldworker to adopt an objectifying and dehumanising relationship to the subjects studied, not unlike the naturalist watching an experiment. He was followed by anthropologists such as Stoller (1989) and Okely (1994), who sought to escape anthropology's ocularcentrism by developing sensuous approaches towards ethnographic understanding. Stoller, for example, devoted a whole chapter to arguing that there was a need for anthropologists to reorient their senses away from the visualism of the West and towards 'the smells, tastes and textures of the land, the people, and the food' (1989: 29). Likewise, Howes (1991), in an edited volume about the senses, proclaimed that a whole new subfield of anthropology, which he labelled the 'anthropology of the senses', was developing.[1] While he considered this to be primarily concerned with how modalities of sensory experience vary from one culture to the next, he also expressed the hope that 'the wisdom gained by *plunging* into the realm of the non-visual senses and exploring how the possibilities of awareness contained within these senses have been exploited by others can help to *liberate* us from the hegemony which sight has for so long exercised over our own culture's social, intellectual, and aesthetic life' (1991: 4, his emphasis).

Yet, one is led to wonder whether this recent commitment in anthropology to making a case against vision is really as comprehensively proven as it seems. I do not believe so, and in this chapter I shall argue from the position that there is nothing inherently problematic about making vision our model for knowing and understanding the world. In fact, through the arguments and the evidence presented, my hope is to re-establish some of anthropology's lost confidence in vision and visual forms of experience and knowledge. My point is not to return to ocularcentrism, which takes the knowledge inherent in vision for granted, but rather to re-examine the kind of knowledge that this sensory modality permits or encourages. In particular, I shall draw attention to the fact that vision's capacity '*to have at a distance*' (Merleau-Ponty 1964: 166) allows for a certain withholding or non-giving of the self, which is of paramount importance to 'liminal' modes of being-in-the-world, such as those of the Siberian Yukaghir hunter and the ethnographic field researcher, each of whom strives for assimilation with otherness while in some profound sense remaining the same. The recent attempt to turn away from vision and depose it from its former privileged status within anthropological thought and discourse is therefore highly controversial and should not go unchallenged.

Previous Studies: 'seeing as actual practice'

I am not the first anthropologist to re-examine, and indeed to call into question, the current tendency to discard vision as an objectifying sense that naturally exposes and dominates the world around us. Thus, Ingold (2000), in an important article about the senses, has suggested that modern society's orientation towards surveying and dominating objects rests not so much on its supposed favouring of vision, but rather on a certain narrow conception of thought: 'Evidently, the primacy of vision cannot be held to account for the objectification of the world. Rather the reverse; it is through its co-option in the service of a particular modern project of objectification that vision has been reduced to a faculty of pure, disinterested reflection …' (2000: 235).

He goes on to argue that to take the charge against vision seriously, one would have to show that seeing as *actual practice* harbours within itself a tendency towards objectification, surveillance and display of power. Yet, such an attempt would be destined to fail because: '*What* we see is inseparable from *how* we see, and how we see is always a function of the practical activity in which we are engaged' (Ingold 2000: 260, his emphasis). In other words, according to Ingold, there is no such thing as seeing in the singular, but rather an indefinite number of ways of seeing, all of which depend on the type of practical relationship that we establish with things and people around us. Thus, what his assessment draws attention to is the common flaw running through most of the criticisms of ocularcentrism, which is the attempt in these writings to divorce the study of vision from people's actual practices of looking.

In a recent study of cattle breeders in northern Italy, Grasseni (2004: 1–15) reinforces this point. Thus, she argues that among the herders, vision plays a paramount part, but it is 'not as a disembodied "overview" from nowhere, but as a capacity to look in a certain way as a result of training' (ibid. 1). She labels this mode of looking 'skilled vision' and contrasts it with the intellectual discourse surrounding vision as being distant, cold and disinterested.

Likewise, Grimshaw (2001), in her treatment of ways of seeing in modern anthropology, presents the argument that differentiating modes if not kinds of vision may be a more useful strategy for examining the ideological, epistemological and representational implications of anthropology's ocularcentric paradigm: 'There are a number of kinds of anthropological visuality or ways of seeing making up the modern [anthropological] project. The category "observation" is only one of these; and even this ... may mean something different from the stereotypes enshrined in much critical discourse' (2001: 7). She thus sets out to deconstruct the principles in terms of which the question of the hegemony of vision in anthropology has been formulated, opposing the notion that it is possible to define vision in some unified or essentialist way. At the same time, she attempts to flaunt and subvert the character of this mode of vision by showing us ways of seeing in anthropology freed from, and opposed to, the objectifying gaze of the detached observer.

While I completely agree with Ingold's argument that vision is in an important sense *practical*, inseparably bound up with the type of activity in which we are engaged and with his and the other scholars' attempt to re-embed vision within its primary context of people's actual perceptual engagement with the world around them, I am nevertheless led to wonder whether this then implies that seeing exists only as it is instantiated in activity itself, and that nothing can be said about vision per se or about the particular mode of world-relation this sensory modality permits or encourages. Surely there must be more to vision than the indefinite number of practical contexts in which it is employed?

I take this point from Leder (1990: 29), who has argued that variations in our use of the senses 'are possible only within, and are limited by, the common structure of the body... upon which all cultures must build'. Could it be, then, that we can uncover certain invariants in visual experience that, instead of being totally arbitrary, remain relatively constant throughout the range of practical and cultural variations? Although one should be cautious with such a line of argument and acknowledge that our sensory modalities and interpretations are always already deeply shaped by cultural practices, I find it tempting to follow Lender's suggestion that our body's fundamental anatomy and physiology delineate and suggest the modes of usage to which the different sensory modalities are put. Accordingly, in this article I shall venture to take the analytical framework of 'seeing as actual practice' to a yet more fundamental level of analysis by drawing attention to the similar ways in which vision is put to use as a kind of defence mechanism against the dissolution of the self by two so very different cultural groups as Siberian Yukaghir hunters and social anthropologists.

Merleau-Ponty and Vision

I draw my main theoretical inspiration from the phenomenologically inspired philosophy of Merleau-Ponty, who, as Jay writes, attempted to 'reaffirm the nobility of vision', but whose work was 'cut short by his untimely death' and was therefore 'never satisfactory completed' (1993: 160).[2] Merleau-Ponty's body of work is by no means easy to interpret in any definitive manner. His final work, in particular, *The Visible and the Invisible* (2000 [1968]), is not only highly fragmentary and obscure, but effectively incomplete. Nonetheless, what I single out as its most illuminating insight in relation to my argument is his assertion that '*to see is to have at a distance.*' I take this as the founding statement of my approach to vision. What it means is that our distance from things is not an obstacle to seeing but its precondition. It is through our distance from things that we, as seeing persons, can become close to them. In vision, therefore, distance and proximity are not mutually exclusive, but rather imply one another. Merleau-Ponty rightly says that they coincide (2000: 135).

This insight is, I shall argue, of particular importance for our understanding of practices in which people steer a difficult course between transcending difference and maintaining identity. Thus, I shall show that the basic theme of self-and-other in ethnographic fieldwork is particularly dependent on the unique capacity of vision to bring us into contact with others by concretely making a distance between our embodiment and theirs. Yet, in developing my argument, I shall not simply address the experience of fieldwork itself, but problematise it through the hunting activity of the Yukaghirs, a small Siberian indigenous group among whom I have conducted years of fieldwork. Rather like the ethnographic field researcher, they attempt to transcend the self–other interface by establishing spaces of shared bodily and sensory experience. For the Yukaghirs, however, the 'significant' other is not a fellow human being but an animal to be hunted and killed for food. Nonetheless, I shall show that the Yukaghir hunters, too, must rely on vision to establish the right proportion between distance and proximity in relation to their prey. In the following sections, I shall devote myself to the Yukaghir ethnography, and at the end of the article return to discuss what I take to be analogies between their use of vision and that of the anthropologist.

The Principles of Yukaghir Hunting

The Yukaghirs, along with many other hunting peoples in Siberia and the Americas, have developed a highly complex ontology of seeing and knowing, recently described as 'perspectivism' (Viveiros de Castro 1998).[3] This is the conception 'according to which the world is inhabited by different sorts of subjects or persons, human or non-human, which see reality from distinct points of view' (ibid. 469). However, these are not alternative points of view of the same world, but rather result from a carrying-over of the same point of view into alternative realities. Thus, every species, within its own sphere, sees the world in the same way – that is, in the same way that human beings do. But *what* each one sees is different, and depends on the kind of body it has. Hence the remarkable notion that:

> Humans see humans as humans, animals as animals and spirits (if they see them) as spirits; however animals (predators) and spirits see humans as animals (as prey) to the same extent that animals (as prey) see humans as spirits or as animals (predators). By the same token, animals and spirits see themselves as humans: they perceive themselves as (or become) anthropomorphic beings when they are in their own houses or villages, and they experience their own habits and characteristics in the form of culture. (Viveiros de Castro 1998: 470)

In this perspectival universe, in which all living creatures see themselves as humans and all others are seen as either predators or prey, hunting becomes an exercise in trickery, in which the hunter undergoes a long process of preparations by which his body is transformed into the image of an elk, which is by far the most important prey animal of the Yukaghirs (Willerslev 2004a; 2004b). The elk then comes to see the hunter not as an evil spirit or a predator, but as a harmless friend and a member of its own species. Accordingly, Yukaghir hunters visit the sauna on the evening before leaving for the forest, where, instead of using soap, they wipe themselves with whisks from birch trees. They say that the elk recognises the attractive smell of birch and does not flee, but comes closer to the hunter. Moreover, small children, who are said to have a particularly strong human odour, are kept away from hunters. At home, affection for children is expressed by sniffing. Parents apply their noses to the napes of their children's necks and inhale their odour. However, when a hunter sets off for the forest, he rarely embraces his offspring. This is in order to avoid contamination with their odour. Transcending the human–non-human interface is also evident in the Yukaghirs' general obsession with exploring animal behaviour. I once witnessed a hunter eating willow bark. When I asked him why he did this, he explained that it was in order to find out what the favourite food of the elk tasted like (Willerslev 2001: 46).

Thus, hunters draw on the full range of bodily senses in constructing correspondences between themselves and their prey. Yet, in so doing, they run the risk of being carried away by their animal identity and undergoing an irreversible metamorphosis. The Yukaghirs talk about this as the prey animal taking on a 'human appearance', because, according to the principles of perspectivism, this is how all beings that share the same corporality are believed to see one another. Thus, Yukaghirs tell anxiety-provoking stories in which hunters begin to see their prey as fellow human beings and follow them back to their households, never to return to their ordinary sphere of existence.

It follows from this that although the hunter identifies with the animal, taking on its behaviour, senses and sensibilities as though they were his own, the distance between himself and his prey, between his experience and that of the animal, must never vanish altogether. Consequently, the hunter must retain a certain element of self-awareness or reflexivity in order to safeguard himself against any absolute identification with his prey. It is, so to speak, this very element of distance that the hunter establishes between himself and the animal, which allows him to enter into its life-world and undergo vicarious experiences. Without this distance, proximity between the two would simply be impossible, as the hunter would collapse into the animal and undergo an irreversible metamorphosis. For the hunter, therefore, proximity is possible only when preceded by distance. (Figure 1.1 shows hunters with a dead elk.)

But what is it that allows for this strikingly necessary distance that makes it possible for the hunter to take on an animal's identity and experience its life-world? This ability, I shall argue, is in a fundamental manner bound up with his capacity for vision. However, to sustain this claim we will need to inquire more closely into sight as a discrete sense that possesses a particular manner of access to the world and to the self-awareness of the seeing subject.

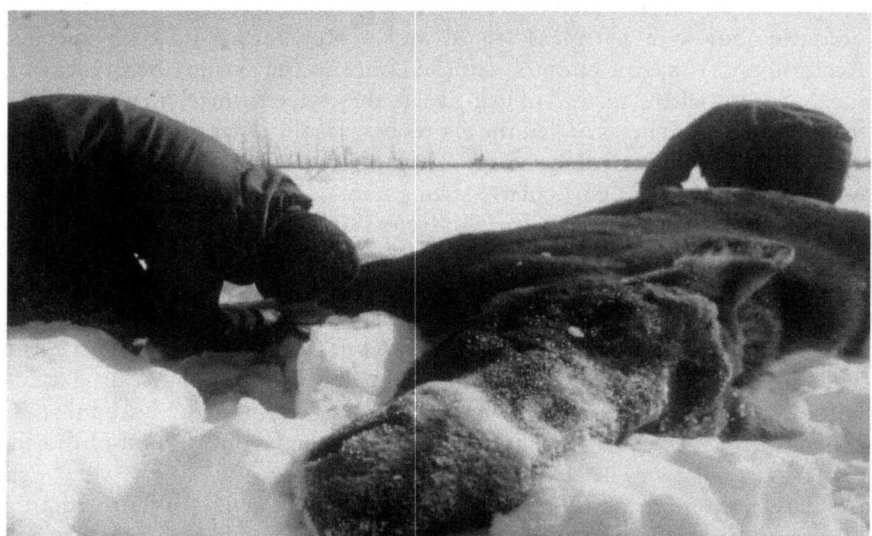

Figure 1.1 *Hunters with dead elk. (Photo: Rane Willerslev)*

Vision and the Other Senses

Merleau-Ponty tells us that '*to see is to have at a distance*' (1964: 166). What he is referring to is the fact that we cannot open our eyes to things without distancing ourselves from them. 'Separation is the price of vision' (de Certeau 1983: 26). However, this distance is not an obstacle to seeing, but rather its precondition. It is, so to speak, because of the distance we have from things that we, as seeing persons, are near to them. If we get too close to the visible object, both the object and our vision disappear. When our eyes come too near to a thing, we experience blurring, then blindness. Thus, our look takes things up and makes them visible only from a certain distance.

This principle of perception contrasts with the so-called proximity senses: smell, taste and touch. None of these modalities gains, but all lose, through distance (Jonas 2001 [1966]: 150). The sense of touch, for example, requires the toucher to be in direct contact with the object touched; taste further implicates the subject, as the object must be internalised in order for it to be accessible to taste. As such, taste involves an experience of undifferentiation in which 'inside' and 'outside', 'me' and 'not-me', blur into confusion and merge.

As for hearing: although, like sight, it requires a distance and suffers from over-closeness, we are inclined to hear sound 'in' the ear, rather than situating it in space. The distance of hearing, therefore, is not set opposite the listener, but streams towards and into him. This is in accord with Zuckerlandl, who formulates the difference between vision and hearing as one between the experience of a world 'out there', and that of a world coming 'from-out-there-toward-me-and-through-me' (1956: 368). Also Ong points to precisely this difference, when he argues that sound gets inside us and touches the innermost surfaces of our being in a way that is impossible for sight, which puts the observer at a remove from the object:

> Whereas sight situates the observer outside what he views, at a distance, sound pours into the hearer ... [Thus] you can immerse yourself in hearing, in sound. There is no way to immerse yourself similarly in sight. (1982: 71)

As a matter of fact, we know from experience that watching a horror film with the sound turned down is not at all scary. However, even with our face turned away from the television screen, we may find it impossible to escape the impression of the film's creepy music. The following passage from Straus also touches upon this theme:

> We can flee from something which is visible in the distance. But that which is heard – be it sound or word – has already taken hold of us; in hearing we have already heard. (1963: 378)

Our auditory experience, then, is essentially intimate, one of immersion, and so the 'out there' quality that we experience in vision is replaced by a feeling of impact that calls one back to the proximate co-presence of the body with its object, similar to that of the senses of smell, touch and taste.

Consequently, the difference between vision and the other senses is essentially a difference in the intensity of the contact and the closeness of things in relation to our bodies. With regard to the non-visual senses, we merge with the world in a manner that is much more direct and intimate than is the case with vision, whose quality lies in a lack of proximity between the object of perception and the body of the percipient.[4] Indeed, Jonas (2001: 149) encapsulates this point eloquently when he writes: 'the best view is by no means the closest view; to get the proper view we take the proper distance'.

Seeing and Being Seen

It is also the element of distance inherent in vision that, in a fundamental way, allows for radical reflection; i.e. allows us to become, in a sense, the 'objects' of our own gaze. Such modalities as taste, touch and smell make less dramatic contributions to conscious self-awareness, since these modalities lack the distance between subject and object by which the subject precisely recognises himself as a separate being.[5] With regard to vision, in contrast, I have described how to see a thing is *not* to coincide blindly with it or to be it. Rather, the seeing of a phenomenon requires a *distance*, a space between the 'here' of the seer and the 'there' of the phenomenon, and – this is the key point – this distance allows the subject not only to be aware of the visible world but also to be in a fundamental way aware of his own visibility, his own activity of seeing. As Merleau-Ponty writes: 'The enigma is that my body simultaneously sees and is seen. That which looks at all things can also look at itself and recognise, in what it sees, the "other side" of its power of looking. It sees itself seeing ... ' (1964: 162).

Let me explain the meaning of this passage. Our commonsense understanding of vision tells us that we are located where our eyes are. In a literal sense, our commonsense view is egocentric: the world is centred upon the perceiver. But Merleau-Ponty argues that we need to give up this subject-centred view of vision. In reality, the single act of looking is in fact twofold, entailing not only seeing but also being seen. What he suggests by this is not just the trivial point that we are sometimes seen by others; his more interesting (and obscure) claim is that our vision is not only to be understood as a one-way directedness towards the world, but is reflected back towards its own embodiment; its own activity of seeing. In the passage most frequently cited in relation to this point, he quotes a painter's comments: 'In a forest, I have felt many times over that it was not I who was looking at the forest. I felt ... that it was rather the trees that were looking at me' (1964: 167). This experience is entirely familiar to the Koyukon, an indigenous group of hunters, living in the boreal forest of Alaska, who, according to their ethnographer, Nelson, 'live in a world that watches, in a forest of eyes. A person moving through nature – however wild, remote, even desolate the place may be – is never truly alone. The surroundings are aware, sensate, personified' (1983: 14).[6]

The ultimate source of this sensation of being watched is, however, not grounded in the absurd thought that the trees and other things we see also see us in return, thus imputing consciousness and vision to inanimate things. Rather, the trees see us in a manner comparable to that with which a mirror sees us: they reverse the dominant and 'natural' directedness of our vision towards the world back towards its origin in the subject of vision. In this manner, they define a point of view on us that renders us visible to ourselves. When we experience this mirror-sense of vision, we understand that we are visible, precisely because we are seeing. Our seeing returns upon us through the things we see and ultimately leads to our self-recognition as both seeing subjects and objects of seeing. The point to stress here is that our vision not only provides us with fundamental access to the world, but also provides us with fundamental access to ourselves. Indeed, we might say that there is *depth reflexivity* built into vision, which is rooted in the fact that all seeing is doubled with the being seen.[7]

The Hunter's 'double perspective'

If we now turn our attention back to the Yukaghir hunter, who attempts to become sensorially immersed in the life-world of his prey, but must avoid the confusion of total participation, I shall show that he relies on precisely this self-reflexive or mirror-sense of vision to secure the right proportion between distance and proximity in relation to his prey.

When approaching an elk, the hunter wears wooden skis, covered underneath with smooth skin from the leg of an elk, so as to imitate the sound of the animal when moving in snow. In addition, he moves his body like an elk: from side to side in a waddling manner. Provided that the hunter's mimetic performance is convincing, vivid and alive, the elk will leave its hiding place between the trees and bushes and begin to walk towards him, apparently taking him for one of its own kind rather than a human hunter. The two parties will thus approach one another with each doing what the other is doing – that is, each imitating the actions of the other.

The point to stress is that during this situation of mutual mimicry, the hunter must act simultaneously within two motivational spaces, which we might term 'the space of predatory mastery' and 'the space of animal imitation'. The first has to do with the hunter's intention to kill the prey animal, the second with his need to take on its movements and sensory attributes in order to fulfil that intention. The hunter, we might say, acts with a dual nature: he is both hunter and animal. To act in between these two identities is a highly complex task. If he allows his intentions as a hunter to show through his actions, the elk will run away or even attack him. If, on the other hand, he allows his intentions to merge with his bodily movements (which are those of an elk) he will surrender to the perspective of the animal and transform into it. The hunter thus needs to be aware not only of the prey animal seeing him, but *also* of himself seeing prey, to ensure that his perspective is neither that of a hunter nor that of the animal, but somewhere in between, or both at once. In other words, the success of the hunter rests in his ability to maintain a 'double perspective', that of seeing and being seen: seeing the elk as elk (as does a human hunter) along with seeing himself as elk (as seen by the elk he sees).

Hunters express this duality or doubling of perspectives though a series of metaphors. They say that if they see the elk as 'big meat', i.e. as an object to be killed and consumed, it implies that there is no contact at all with the animal, and it will therefore flee. If, on the other hand, a hunter sees the elk as a human being, it means that he himself has surrendered to the single perspective of the prey animal and transformed into it, which is something to be avoided at all costs. For hunters, the right proportion between distance and proximity is thus a perspective in which the animal appears as neither human nor animal, but somewhere in between, or both at once. This notion is strikingly revealed in hunters' narratives, in which the hunter encounters prey that takes on the guise of a human being but retains some of its original species qualities. Bear-man, for example, is said to be recognisable by his jog-trot way of moving, while elk- and reindeer-man tend to leave tracks in the shape of hooves (Willerslev 2004a: 634–35). Among Yukaghir hunters, all techniques and skills of hunting are directed towards this single moment when distance and proximity coincide in a double perspective, when human and non-human, self and other, lose their polarity and swim in and out of focus. This is also the moment at which the animal surrenders to the illusion that what it sees is not an evil spirit or a predator, but a fellow human, and 'gives itself up' to the hunter.

What we might conclude from this, then, is that for Yukaghir hunters, vision is important, not simply as a means of world-disclosure, but also as a defence mechanism against metamorphosis or the dissolution of the self. That is to say, while hunting for the Yukaghirs is a total bodily experience, involving all of the senses, not just vision, as means of comprehending the life-world of their prey, during the critical moment when hunter and elk encounter one another in a situation of face-to-face mimicry and where their bodies tend to blend to a point that makes them of the same kind, the hunter relies fully on vision to safeguard himself against merging with the animal and undergoing an irreversible metamorphosis.

But why this key role played by vision as a mode of self-preservation? As already pointed out, this is essentially rooted in the fact that vision sets a distance between subject and world that allows for a kind of depth reflexivity. In all the other senses, this distance is either lacking or in some way limited. We are, for example, so absorbed in our own smell that we can hardly smell it, just as our tongue cannot taste itself for pure taste. The distance of vision, in contrast, allows the hunter to 'see himself seeing' – that is, it allows him not only to share the bodily texture, senses and sensibilities of his prey, but also to be reflexively aware of himself as standing apart from it as a subject with a perspective of his own (and a human one at that). Thus, the distance of vision uniquely provides the hunter with a deep reflexive self-awareness that the other senses do not allow for, enabling him to secure boundaries, to distinguish himself, and preserve his human personhood.

Figure-on-a-background

With these observations in mind, let us turn to the question of the relationship of vision to objectification and power. Is there in vision an inherent tendency to expose and dominate the world around us? Numerous intellectuals from many different camps have put forward this claim (cf. Jay 1994). The following statement by Irigaray conflates many of the hostilities to vision expressed by other critics: 'More than any other sense, the eye objectifies and it masters. It sets a distance, and maintains a distance. In our culture the predominance of the look over smell, taste, touch and hearing has brought about an impoverishment of bodily relations' (Irigaray 1978 quoted in Jay 1994: 493).

Yet, one wonders what it is that leads so many distinguished minds to suppose that naturally encoded in vision is a tendency to objectify and master whatever stands before it. And how can my account of vision provide a tool for both criticising this suggestion and recognising its points of validity?

Again, I shall begin my enquiry by turning to Merleau-Ponty, who in his early work, *Phenomenology of Perception*, states: 'it is necessary to put the surroundings in abeyance the better to see the object, and to lose in background what one gains in focal figure' (1998 [1962]: 67). Here, he is drawing heavily upon Gestalt theory and its investigations into the phenomenon of sight. For Gestalt theory, the most basic unit of perceptual experience is that of figure-on-a-background. What this means is basically that the seeing *of* something is invariably the making of a *choice* of what within our visual field must be backgrounded so that something can be perceived in the foreground. In other words, what constitutes visual experience is a dialectic of vagueness and clarity: unthematised or amorphous background and explicit, well-defined figure, to speak in the terms of Gestalt psychology. The important thing to note here is that, although figure and background are reversible correlates in vision – what was figure can become background and vice versa – they are never equivalent in existence: the figure is always the object and value marked against the ground that is the field or unthematised background of vision (Sobchack 1992: 71). As Merleau-Ponty writes: 'One object cannot show itself without concealing others' (1998: 68). We arrive in this way at the notion of the *absolute* object or, as it is sometimes called, the 'strong Gestalt': 'For the Gestalt to be unified and bright – a so-called "strong Gestalt" – all this varied background must become progressively empty and unattractive' (Perls, Hefferline and Goodman 1951, quoted in Levin 1988: 81).

It is with this interplay of figure and ground in mind, polarising, as it does, visual experience into the extremes of gain and loss, strong and weak, full and empty, that Merleau-Ponty (1998: 316) in his early writings suggests that vision pushes objectification further than any of the other senses, for according to the principles of the strong Gestalt, seeing must always be sharply focused, absolutely clear and fixed on its object. There must be nothing hidden, nothing ambiguous, nothing beyond its focal point. As such, vision is fulfilled by what can only be called its 'objectification' of the world – an inherent orientation towards a direct focus on objects that are present, available and masterable (Levin 1988: 74).

The Coming into Being of the Visible

However, I should like to question the supposed universality and necessity of this depiction of vision. While it may be accurate that in the realm of everydayness, vision tends to take the form of figure-on-a-background, there are nevertheless other ways for us to experience the interplay between withdrawing and bringing forth, concealment and unconcealment. I shall illustrate this by returning to the ethnography of the Yukaghirs. For them, any category of physical thing has another modality of being, which they identify as the '*ayibii*,' meaning 'shadow' in their native language. This is what we would call the soul of the thing. Yet, it is not understood as something altogether immaterial, as in our Christian discourse, but rather as an ambiguous combination of spirit and substance. As the name 'shadow' suggests, the *ayibii* resides on the threshold of the visible: it is something visible, yet without being *as such* an actual 'thing' or 'object' (Figure 1.2). As with shadows and reflections, which are themselves not present as objects within our field of vision, but rather hide themselves in making the objects visible by deepening, intensifying and enriching our field of visibility, the *ayibii* tends not to show itself directly to the 'profane' eye, but is said to underlie the visible as its vital or animating principle.

Whenever I asked the Yukaghirs if the *ayibii* appears in any particular form or shape, they frequently explained that whatever entity it belongs to – a human, animal or inanimate object – it would take the same human manifestation, but being like a silhouette in having no details, clothing or features. Why this human form? This is because the *ayibii* defines a prototype of being: an anonymous or general look that precedes and underlies any distinction of perspectives. Thus, in Siberia and the Americas it is a widely held belief that in mythical times, not only humans but also non-humans held a human form and lived and behaved like humans (Bogoras 1904–1909: 283; Brightman 1993: 40; Nelson 1983: 16; Viveiros de Castro 1998: 471–71). At

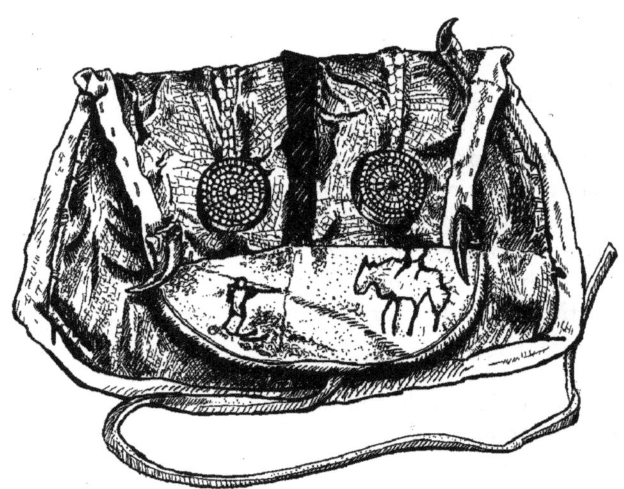

Figure 1.2 *Hunter's container for sewing materials made from swans' feet.* On the front, the hunter's encounter with an elk is depicted. On the back of the animal sits its 'invisible' counterpart, its *ayibii*. (Artwork: Marie Carsten Pedersen)

some point, certain humans died as a result of fighting, by which process they lost their human bodily attributes and became physically distinct as animals, plants and other natural entities with species perspectives of their own. However, since seeing *as such* is a power of the soul, animals and other non-humans continue to see themselves as humans see themselves, but *what* they see is different because their bodies, which are the origin of particular perspectives, are different from those of humans. It follows that: 'The common point of reference for all beings is not humans as a species but rather humanity as a condition' (Descola 1986: 120). 'It has the evident connexion with the idea of animal clothing hiding a common spiritual "essence" and with the issue of the general meaning of perspectivism' (Viveiros de Castro 1998: 472).

Above all, it is the shaman who, through bodily transformations, is capable of assuming the 'infra-human' perspective of other beings. However, laypeople also have, to various degrees, such access. Thus, we have seen how the hunter, when mimicking his prey, replaces his profane vision with a 'double perspective'. It is a mode of seeing, attuned to detecting the intertwining and coming into being of things (as during their creation in mythical times), rather than the things in their clear and fixed visibility or objectness: animals in the process of becoming human; self in the process of becoming other, and so forth. Thus, the hunter sees the formation of 'figures' that, however, are never completed, but remain on the threshold between figure and ground, unconcealment and concealment, visibility and invisibility in a liminal or in-between state of being. Hunters express this when saying that while mimicking prey they not only see the (visible) animal but also its (invisible) human double, its *ayibii*. As already described, the two *co*-appear in the hunter's double perspective (as in Figure 1.2 above).

Also Merleau-Ponty (1964), in his later work, recognises this 'wild' capacity of vision to transcend the rigid dichotomy of figure and ground. For him, the painter is one for whom profane vision is not enough. To paint the profoundly visible, the painter must practise a 'magical theory of vision' (ibid. 166) that uncovers its premises: the ground of the visible within vision. Thus, the painter 'interrogates [the world] with his gaze' (ibid. 167), which does not rest on the familiar forms or figures that everyday vision has time and again constituted, but rather actively searches for the latent visibility from which such figures emerge:

> Light, lighting, shadows, reflections, color, all the objects of his quest are not together real objects; like ghosts, they have only visual existence. In fact they exist only on the threshold of profane vision; they are not seen by everyone. The painter's gaze asks them what they do to suddenly cause something to be and be this thing, what they do to compose this worldly talisman and to make us see the visible. (ibid. 166)

Common for both the hunter and the painter is that their principal medium is sight. Indeed, at their most rigorous, both the hunter and painter practise a kind of phenomenological *epoché* (bracketing) as a means for vision to free itself from the presuppositions of everyday common sense and gain access to the visible world and its essential forms as they actually come into existence. By enquiring into the nature of the way things become visible in vision, they experience how seeing turns around and comes back as though it came from the thing seen. That is, they come to realise how seeing is continuous with being seen and that one could not be without the other. Indeed, this is what they point to when repeatedly insisting that not only do they look at the world, but also the world looks back at them. For the hunter and painter, a reciprocal dimension is therefore always already in operation in vision. Thus, rather than objectifying the world, their vision personifies it; it makes them something for the world to look at.

Vision, Mimesis and Seduction

But what about power? Although the hunter's gaze is not one that strives towards direct focus on objects and total visibility, his activity of hunting nevertheless involves an exercise of power, killing the animal as its ultimate aim. Of crucial importance here is that seeing, as Yukaghir hunters practise it, rests on a principle of mimesis.[8] The hunter undergoes a long process of transformation by means of which his body is shaped into the image of an elk. This in turn makes the animal suspend its disbelief, its inherent hostility towards him, and 'give itself up' to him. Thus, it is not that the hunter forces the animal to submission against its will. Rather, its compliance is secured through what might best be described as a process of 'seduction'. Gebauer and Wulf have noted that: 'Seduction depends on lending form; the seducer's weapon is an image ... As soon as the object of seduction becomes fascinated by this ... image she falls under the power of the seducer ... *Only because the object of seduction desires herself does she let herself be seduced*' (1995: 213; my emphasis).

Thus, the success of the seducer rests on his ability to create an image of the seduced – which, however, is *not* an exact image of how she experiences herself, but rather an ideal representation, a fantasy image of what she could become.[9] Seduction is in this sense inherently narcissistic. It is rooted in the attraction of like to like, in the mimetic exaltation of one's own image, or rather an ideal mirage of resemblance. Indeed, this seems to be the reason why the Yukaghir hunter's fur clothing traditionally had to be carefully and beautifully made. When imitating his prey, he would set in motion an ideal reflection of the animal, exposing as 'exterior' or visible what in reality is 'interior' or invisible: the infra-human perspective of the animal. Thus, what the elk would see in the hunter, the unique object of its attraction, was in fact its *own* seductive, charming self, its lovable self-image – that is, its *ayibii*. The animal, therefore, could not escape this illusory image, but would be compelled to 'embrace' it mimetically. Even today, parts of the hunters' dress are often highly decorated with coloured bands and beadwork (see Figure 1.3). Also, their sheath knives are beautifully ornamented with metalwork. Hunters say that the animal may be so pleased by what it sees that it 'gives itself up to them.'

But then, what is the difference between the hunter's mode of seeing and that of the elk, and is it only the latter that falls victim to the trick of mimicry?

The first point to stress is that although the hunter imitates the elk as if he himself were an elk, this does not mean that the two merge into a state of fusion. While the animal's perspective is encompassed or nested within the hunter's perspective, there is no absolute unity or identity between them. Indeed, this fission or non-coincidence of perspectives is what I have tried to capture when talking about the hunter's 'double perspective', which allows him to see the elk as elk (as does a human person), along with seeing himself as elk (as seen by the elk he sees). Thus, we can say that the hunter moves *inbetween* perspectives, not surrendering to the perspective of a 'single' viewpoint. It is precisely this duality that makes his 'mimetic gaze' such a deadly weapon, because it allows him to take on the viewpoint of his prey, while still remaining a human person with the intention of killing it.

The elk, in contrast, becomes so absorbed in what it sees (its own illusory self-image) that it literally surrenders to the narcissism of a 'single' viewpoint. It finds itself in the hunter and wants to join with him. But in so doing, it violates the strikingly necessary distance of vision and experiences a disturbing disorientation. I have already described how our vision must remain at a distance from the visible world, because otherwise both the visible world and our vision disappear. Vision, therefore, is contact that includes distance; loss of vision is contact without distance. Thus, when the distance of vision is removed, as when the elk grows too close to the hunter, blindness occurs: everything turns into a mass of undifferentiated experience in which inside and outside, self and other, collapse into one, thereby making seeing impossible.

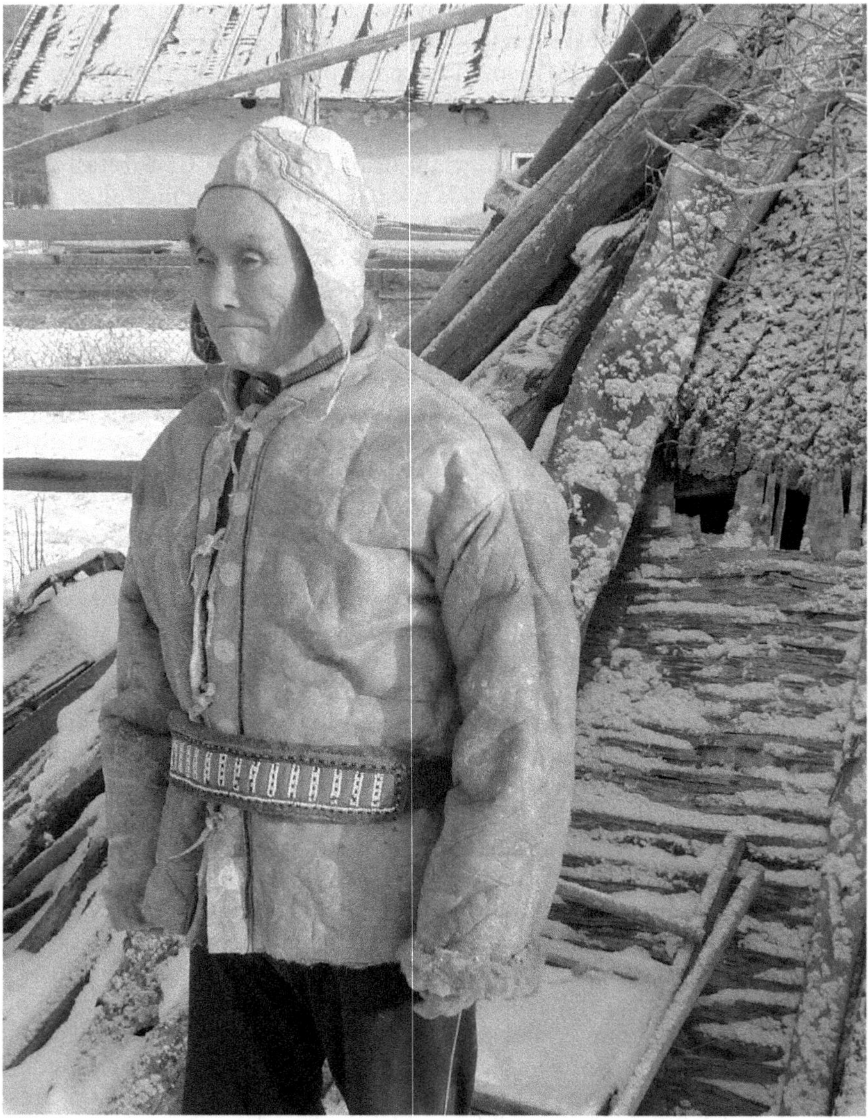

Figure 1.3 *Yukaghir dressed in traditional hunting clothing.* (Photo: Uffe R. Christensen)

The Yukaghirs talk about this as the animal having an innate desire to re-establish the original order of things – an order which, as already described, was characterised by an indistinction of perspectives, a 'seeing in general' (which is the same as no seeing or blindness). Yet, such return to an initial state would mean transforming back into mythical existence, from which people have estranged themselves with such great effort. Thus, hunters say that they must kill the animal before its human bodily appearance is ever completed. Only in overcoming the animal on its way to regaining its humanity can the existing world with its manifold of perspectives be sustained.

The Power to Differentiate

Although the mimetic gaze of the hunter gives him power over his prey, it is a power that is relative and dangerously unstable. I have already described how the hunter may fall victim to his own mimetic tricks and transform into an animal, never to return to his ordinary sphere of existence. Furthermore, not only human hunters but also non-human hunters make use of mimicry as a means of deceiving their prey. Thus, one finds a whole series of stories in which members of the giant cannibal tribe, 'Mystical-Old-People', turn themselves into nice-looking lads to seduce Yukaghir women and eat them. These cannibalistic non-humans call their intended human victims their 'elk' and 'reindeer', thus they address and experience human beings as their animal prey, just as the human hunter does his prey (Jochelson 1926: 302–3).

Hence, it is not that humans are seen as more clever or powerful than non-humans. All beings hold the same capacity for imitation, seduction and deception. Rather, what defines power in the Yukaghir universe, where all parties act as mimetic doubles of each other and where the various boundaries between self and other are permeable and easily crossed, is the ability *not* to confuse analogy with identity. To exercise power is to steer a difficult course between transcending difference and maintaining identity: to see the world from the perspectives of various others, yet avoiding total participation and confusion. Indeed, this is why the Yukaghirs attach such tremendous importance to vision as a source of power, because the fact is that to '*have at a distance*' of vision is both having *and* distantiation. As seer, one may therefore enter into relations with see-able others and be transformed, but without necessarily losing oneself in the process. Surely, this is 'the paradoxical enigmatic "madness" of vision' (Jay 1994: 314–15).

Conclusion: the Significance of Vision for Anthropology

It was Malinowski (1922: 25) who first claimed that anthropology was concerned with an understanding of other cultures from the 'native's point of view'. Although his observationalist stance implied 'observation at the closest possible *distance*', the element of distantiation has since then largely been neglected in favour of a very strong, almost obsessive fixation on overcoming the self--other interface as the precondition essential for acquiring anthropological understanding. Hastrup summarises this quest for the sublation of distance very well, when she writes:

> The necessity of a close association with the natives ... has been expressed in different ways according to paradigm ... and although it has been claimed that the notion of 'immersion' in the foreign culture is most often totally unwarranted, no anthropologist seems to deny that 'the closer the better.' To 'know' another world, one must associate with the natives, even possibly become one of them, at least temporarily. (1993: 174)

One of the more recent paradigms stressing this need to fully 'negate' differences is the so-called 'anthropology of the senses', whose supporters argue that anthropologists should draw on the full range of bodily senses in an attempt to overcome the distance of the other (Classen 1993; Howes 1991; Okely 1994). Stoller (1989), for example, has argued the need for us to reorient ourselves away from the visualism of the West and towards 'the smells, tastes and textures of the land, the people, and the food [...] letting our senses be penetrated by the world of the other' (ibid. 29, 39). In fact, he is so anxious that 'a person's spatialized "gaze" creates distance', that he can follow his own advice only by learning to hear, rather than to see, as the natives do (ibid. 120).[10]

However, what Stoller and the others, who hold that our quest for anthropological understanding should be animated by a total openness to otherness, seem to miss is that any attempt at proximity quite crucially takes distance as its precondition: it is the distance of persons as distinct from one another that allows us to place ourselves within another's experience. Proximity would be impossible in the absence of distance, because then the experiencer and the experienced would conflate, would become one, thereby making experience of the other impossible. Thus, what anthropology is in search of is not an experience of truly radical proximity, but a type of experience that puts us in contact with others and yet separates us from them, keeping us at a distance. And there is, of course, such an experience, an experience that is grounded in '*the having at a distance*' of vision.

Vision, as I have described, brings us into contact with others by concretely making a distance between our embodiment and theirs. It is, so to say, because of this distance that we as seeing persons are close to them. Thus, distance and proximity are in this case not mutually exclusive but rather imply one another: the eye achieves unity and separation at one and the same time. Indeed, vision is our 'liminal' sense *par excellence* – for what is liminality but literally the 'threshold', the space that both separates and joins spaces? (Schechner 1985: 295). This might explain, or at least accommodate, the fact that anthropology traditionally has been firmly based in vision and visual forms of experience and knowledge, because it is hard to imagine how the world of liminality established in the field would be possible without vision. Only the *'having at a distance'* of vision allows us to be part of an alien reality, while at the same time detaching ourselves from that reality by keeping at a distance.

My point in all of this is not that anthropologists should simply 'look' at the world, ignoring the other modalities, as a means of understanding others. The doctrine of 'synesthesia', one of Merleau-Ponty's (1998: 228–29) long-standing tenets, prohibits us from regarding the various senses as altogether discrete or isolated from one another. All our senses are modalities of perception, and are as such cooperative and commutable. Our sight is, consequently, never just sight – it sees what our hands can touch, our nose can smell, and our tongue can taste. Indeed, all of our non-visual senses are implicated in our vision, and there is no such activity as 'just' looking (Sobchack 1992: 78).[11]

However, there are certain moments in which perception needs to be most fully focused and localised in one of its modalities, when it needs to be dominated and directed by a specific sense. I described how this was the situation with the Yukaghir hunter in his mimetic encounter with the elk, and the same can be said for the anthropologist in the field. For both, their principal medium is and *must* be sight, because only vision offers the possibility of encountering the other 'safely'. Why is this? For the reason that, more than any other sense, vision sets and maintains a distance. The reflexive presence of oneself to oneself occurs only mediated by distance, which is why the *'having at a distance'* of vision uniquely provides us with a sort of depth reflexivity (a seeing that not only sees the world, but turns back upon itself, making itself visible). This self-reflexive or mirror-sense of vision is, as I have shown, strikingly necessary as a kind of defence mechanism against the dissolution of the self in relations where people steer a difficult course between transcending difference and maintaining identity. Thus, although ethnographic fieldwork is a total bodily experience, involving all of the senses and not just vision as a means of understanding others, it is above all due to the primacy of sight that we can share the life-world of others, while still drawing our boundaries and saying: 'I am the other of those others.'

Acknowledgements

For helpful comments, I warmly thank Alberto Corsin Jimenez, Rebecca Empson, Penny Harvey, Anne Line Dalsgaard, Bodil Selmer and Coilín ÓhAiseadha.

Notes

1 The phrase, 'the cultural anthropology of the senses', was first used by the historian Roy Porter in his preface to *The Foul and the Fragrant: Odor and the French Social Imagination*, by Alain Corbin (Porter 1986). However, the anthropology of the senses did not arise as a definite field within anthropology until the late 1980s (Herzfeld 2001: 249).

2 Merleau-Ponty's attempt for a salvation of sight should be understood in relation to Sartre, who in *Being and Nothingness* (1966) described quite vividly the anxiety and tension that can be experienced through the awareness of being looked at. It is impossible here to give a complete summary of his account. Instead, I will try to briefly summarise the main points of contrast between the two accounts. Sartre describes the effect of the look in terms of alienation. To experience the other's look is to experience oneself as no longer belonging to oneself but as belonging as an object in the project of the other. This involves a change in our very existence. We are not normally objects of our own contemplation, in Sartre's view. Rather, we simply live our life without having it as an object of our thoughts. The other's look, however, tears us away from this. Through it we suddenly come to thematise ourselves as an object within the world. Yet, this is not how we habitually experience ourselves to be. To this extent we feel estranged. To Sartre, therefore, we must choose to see or to be seen, to expose the others to our look or to be exposed ourselves. This dialectic is essential to his post-Hegelian account of freedom, where selfhood is depicted as constituted through a power struggle for recognition: a struggle whose purpose it is to remain seeing and not to be reduced to an object of another's vision.

Merleau-Ponty, by contrast, stresses that in order for us to see we must be visible to others. Our own visibility is the very condition of our seeing, and there is therefore no inherent conflict between seeing and being seen. Rather, the two are inextricably bound up together, and one could not be without the other. This, however, does not mean that the seer and the seen coincide in a state of fusion, the seer's total identification with the other. There is, according to Merleau-Ponty, some separation between the two precisely because there is a distance built into vision. This distance, however, does not necessarily lead to objectification and alienation, as Sartre would have it. Quite the opposite, the distance of vision is in fact sociality's precondition: it is what allows us to exchange one another's perspectives. Social relations would be impossible in the absence of distance. Thus, vision, rather than being our antisocial sense *par excellence*, as implied by Sartre, is in fact its foundation. It is by situating the distance of vision as essential to sociality that I believe Merleau-Ponty can be said to rethink its nobility.

3 Besides the Amazon and Siberia, perspectival notions are strikingly apparent among hunting peoples in the Arctic and sub-Arctic, such as the Inuit (Saladin d'Anglure 2001) and the Cree and Ojibwa Indians (Brightman 1993: 41–48; Hallowell 1960: 36: Tanner 1979: 136–37). Moreover, perspectivism is also present among hunting peoples of Southeast Asia, such as the Chewong of the Malay tropical forest (Howell 1996). In a previous article (Willerslev 2004a), I have criticised Viveiros de Castro's outline of perspectivism for dealing with the cosmological order of things rather than with practices, and I have suggested that linking it with 'mimesis' would allow us to treat the perspectival ideas of hunting peoples as practical constructs rather than abstract categories. Having said this, I find it likely that Viverios de Castro's and my different views on perspectivism can at least partly be explained by the fact that his analysis is centred on the world of the shaman while my starting point is the hunter. However, in my view, we might find a plausible grounding (if not origin) of perspectivism in hunting. After all, shamanism is in many of these communities often an extension or elaboration of the hunting process, so that the difference between the hunter and the shaman is one of degree rather than kind. This could also explain why it is, as Viveiros de Castro himself observes, that the dynamics of predator and prey are fundamental to perspectival thinking among shamans (1998: 471).

4 With respect to this, it is interesting to recall a conversation I had with an anthropologist who was studying blind people. She was blindfolded for a prolonged period of time in order to gain a sense of what it is like to be blind, and described this experience to me as feeling as if the world were falling down upon her. This seems to agree with Lusseyran (quoted in Hill 1985: 107), who writes that 'what the blind person experiences in the presence of an object is "pressure"'. Also Hull (1997: 23) in his study of blind people reports precisely this experience, describing the pressure of one's surroundings as being sometimes so intense that one instinctively wants to put a hand up to the face to protect oneself.

5 This point finds support in research on the development of children born blind, which reveals that it takes them significantly longer to appropriate a unified self-image and to subsequently learn the stable use of the pronoun 'I' (Fraiberg and Adelson 1973; quoted in Ver Eecke 1975). Furthermore, even once this appropriation is achieved, blind children's 'postural schema ... [and] image and experience of ... [their bodies] ... vary considerably from that of sighted subjects' (Grosz 1990).

6 For another fascinating account of the perceptual experience of seeing and being seen, see Empson's (2005) article on the Mongolian household chest, where multiple kinship relations are revealed at once, to the viewer as he looks at himself looking at the image revealed in the display.

7 This, however, is not to deny the fact that there is reflexivity build into other senses than sight. In fact, in taking up the issue of reversibility in seeing, Merleau-Ponty (2000 [1968]: 133) explicitly states that he will consider it as a variant of tactile reversibility (one hand touching the other: what is commonly known as 'double sensation'). Yet, in my interpretation of his work, the tactile reversibility is to be understood as the equivalent of what he in his earlier work addresses under the heading of the 'tacit cogito': 'self-consciousness, which is unaware of itself in its fascination with the world' (Dillon 1988: 105). The tacit cogito only becomes explicit 'in those extreme situations in which it is under threat: for example, in the dread of death or in the look of another' (Merleau-Ponty 1968: 404). Thus, the explicit reflexivity, described by Descartes as the act of res cogitas, is intimately linked to vision's reversibility of seeing and being seen. The movement from tactility to vision is therefore the progress from the 'tacit' consciousness of the body to the 'explicit' consciousness of the self.

8 The painter's relationship to the world is also essentially mimetic. Merleau-Ponty tells us that when the artist paints the world, he 'lends' his body to it to bring forth 'a metamorphosis of the visible' (1964: 161). Moreover, just like the hunter, the painter does not force himself onto the world. Rather, there is a sense in which the world 'gives itself up to him': 'The labor of the painter is the birth of expression and the world *call* or *demand this birth* (Johnson 1993: 27: my emhasis). However, in lending his body to the world, the painter also runs the risk of being swallowed up by it. Indeed, this is what happened to Cézanne, Merleau-Ponty's favourite artist. Again and again he lent his body to the Montagne Sainte-Victoire, which he painted year after year from different angles and at diffrerent times of the day and during different seasons. But in the end Cézanne was swallowed up by the very mountain with which he identified: while painting it, he was caught in a huge storm and died.

9 I talk about the elk as a 'she', since the Yukaghirs generally conceptualise the animal as a woman, who 'gives herself up' to the male hunter out of sexual desire for him. In fact, hunters' terminology is replete with symbolic parallels between elk hunting and sexual seduction (Willerslev 2004a).

10 I take this point from Ingold (2000: 252).

11 This, however, does not mean that our senses are equivalent. Each brings with it 'a structure of being that can never be exactly transposed' (Merleau-Ponty 1998: 225). This is why formerly blind people, whose sight has been restored, initially find their predicament so bewildering: tactile experience turns out to be a poor guide to the visual world, not because it is relatively impoverished but because the tactile world is differently structured (ibid. 222–24). Thus, in his doctrine of synesthesia, Merleau-Ponty does not intend to conflate the senses. The senses are united in one body and open onto a unitary world, but to lose one of them is to lose a quality of experience that the remaining senses cannot restore.

References

Bogoras, W. and W. Bogoras, 1904–1909. *The Chukchee, Memoir of the American Museum of Natural History*, ed. F. Boas, Vol. VII, New York: American Museum of Natural History.

Brightman, R. 1993. *Grateful Prey: Rock Cree Human-animal Relationships*. Berkeley, Los Angeles, Oxford: University of California Press.

de Certeau, M. 1983. 'The Madness of Vision', trans. M.B. Smith, Enclitic 7 (1), University of Minnesota.

Classen, C., 1993. *Worlds of Sense: Exploring the Senses in History and Across Cultures*. London and New York: Routledge.

Descola, P. 1986. La Nature Domestique: Symbolism et Praxis dans l'Ecologie des Achuar. Paris: Maison des Science de l'Homme

Dillon, M.C., 1988. *Merleau-Ponty's Ontology*. Evanston: Northwestern University Press.

Empson, R. 2005. 'Separating and Containing People and Things in Mongolia', in *Thinking through Things: Artefacts in Ethnographic Perspective*, eds. A. Henare, M. Holbraad and S. Wastell, London: Cavendish University of London Press.

Fabian, J. 1983. *Time and the Other: How Anthropology Makes its Object*. New York: Columbia University Press.

Gebauer, G. and C. Wulf, 1995. *Mimesis: Culture, Art, Society*, trans. D. Reneau. Berkeley: University of California Press.

Grasseni, C. 2004. 'Skilled Vision: an Apprenticeship in Breeding Aesthetics', *Social Anthropology* 12 (1): 1–15.

Grimshaw, A. 2001. *The Ethnographer's Eye: Ways of Seeing in Modern Anthropology*. Cambridge: Cambridge University Press.

Grosz, E. 1990. *Jacques Lacan: A Feminist Introduction*. London: Routledge.

Hallowell, A.I. 1960. 'Ojibwa Ontology, Behavior and World-view', in Culture in History: Essays in Honor of Paul Radin, ed. S. Dimond. New York: Columbia University Press, 19–52.

Hastrup, K. 1993. 'The Native Voice and the Anthropological Vision', *Social Anthropology/Anthropologie Sociale* 1: 173-–86.

Herzfeld, M. 2001. *Theoretical Practice in Culture and Society*. Blackwell Publishers, UNESCO MOST.

Hill, M.H. 1985. 'Bound to the Environment: Towards a Phenomenology of Sightlessness', in *Dwelling, Place and Environment*, eds. D. Seamon and R. Mugerauer. New York: Columbia University Press, 99–111.

Howell, S. 1996. 'Nature in Culture or Culture in Nature? Chewong Ideas of 'Humans' and Other Species', in *Nature and Society: Anthropological Perspectives*, eds. P. Descola and G. Pàlsson. London: Routledge, 127–44.

Howes, D. 1991. 'Sensory Anthropology', in *The Varieties of Sensory Experience: A Sourcebook in the Anthropology of the Senses*, ed. D. Howes. Toronto: University of Toronto Press, 167–91.

Hull, J. 1997. *On Sight and Insight: A Journey into the World of Blindness*. Oxford: Oneworld Publications.

Ingold, T. 2000. 'Stop, Look and Listen! Vision, Hearing and Human Movement', in T. Ingold, *The Perception of the Environment: Essays in Livelihood, Dwelling and Skill*. London and New York: Routledge, 243–87.

Jay, M. 1994. *Downcast Eyes: the Denigration of Vision in Twentieth-century French Thought*. Berkeley, Los Angeles, London: University of California Press.
—— 1993. 'Sartre, Merleau-Ponty, and the Search for a New Ontology of Sight', in *Modernity and the Hegemony of Vision*, ed. D.M. Levin. Berkeley, Los Angeles, London: University of California Press, 143-85.
Jochelson, W. 1926. *The Yukaghir and the Yukaghized Tungus*, in Memoir of the American Museum of Natural History, ed. F. Boas. New York: American Museum of Natural History.
Johnson, G.A. 1993. 'Ontology and Painting: 'Eye and Mind'', in *The Merleau-Ponty Aesthetics Reader: Philosophy and Painting*, ed. G.A. Johnson. Evanston: Northwestern University Press, 35–55.
Jonas, H. 2001 [1966]. *The Phenomenon of Life*. Chicago: Chicago University Press.
Leder, D. 1990. *The Absent Body*. Chicago and London: The University of Chicago Press.
Levin, D.M. 1988. *The Opening of Vision: Nihilism and the Post-modern Situation*. London: Routledge.
Malinowski, B. 1922. *Argonauts of the Western Pacific*. London: Routledge.
Merleau-Ponty, M., 1964. 'Eye and Mind', in *The Primacy of Perception and Other Essays on Phenomenological Psychology, the Philosophy of Art, History and Politics*, ed. J. Wild. Northwestern University Press, 159-90.
—— 1998 [1962]. *Phenomenology of Perception*, trans. C. Smith. London: Routledge & Kegan Paul.
—— 2000 [1968]. *The Visible and the Invisible*. Evanston: Northwestern University Press.
Nelson, R. 1983. *Make Prayers to the Raven: A Koyukon View of the Northern Forest.* Chicago and London: The University of Chicago Press.
Okely, J. 1994. 'Vicarious and Sensory Knowledge of Chronology and Change: Ageing in Rural France', in *Social Experience and Anthropological Knowledge*, eds. K. Hastrup and P. Hervik. London: Routledge, 45–64.
Ong, W. 1982. *Orality and Literacy: the Technologizing of the Word*. London: Methuen.
Porter, R. 1986. 'Foreword', in A. Corbin, *The Foul and the Fragrant: Odor and the French Social Imagination*, trans. M.L. Kochan, R. Porter and C. Prendergast. Cambridge, Mass: Harvard University Press, v–vii.
Saladin d'Anglure, B. 2001. 'Erotic Dreams, Mystical Kinship, and Shamanism', North Atlantic Studies: Shamanism and Traditional Beliefs 4: 1–2.
Sartre, J.P. 1966. *Being and Nothingness: an Essay on Phenomenological Ontology*, trans. H.E. Barnes. New York: Washington Square Press.
Schechner, R. 1985. *Between Theatre and Anthropology*. Philadelphia: University of Pennsylvania Press.
Sobchack, V. 1992. *The Address of the Eye: a Phenomenology of Film Experience*. Princeton: Princeton University Press.
Stoller, P. 1989. *The Taste of Ethnographic Things: the Senses in Anthropology*. Philadelphia: University of Pennsylvania.
Straus, E. 1963. *The Primary World of Senses: Towards a Philosophical Biology*, trans. J. Needleman. Glencoe: The Free Press of Glencoe.
Tanner, A. 1979. *Bringing Home Animals*. London: Hust.
Ver Eecke, W. 1975. 'The Look, the Body, and the Other', in *Dialogues in Phenomenology*, eds. D. Ihde and R.M. Zaner. The Hague: Martinus Nijoff.

Viveiros de Castro, E., 1998. 'Cosmological Deixis and Amerindian Perspectivism', *Journal of the Royal Anthropological Institute* (N.S.) 4: 469–88.

Willerslev, R. 2001. 'The Hunter as a Human 'Kind': Hunting and Shamanism among the Upper Kolyma Yukaghirs of Siberia', *North Atlantic Studies: Shamanism and Traditional Beliefs*, 4 (1+2): 44–50.

—— 2004a. 'Not Animal, Not-not Animal: Hunting, Imitation and Emphathetic Knowledge among the Siberian Yukaghirs', *The Journal of the Royal Anthropological Institute*, 10 (3): 629–52.

—— 2004b. 'Spirits as "Ready to Hand": a Phenomenological Analysis of Yukaghir Spiritual Knowledge and Dreaming', *Anthropological Theory*, 4 (4): 395–418.

Zuckerlandl, V. 1956. *Sound and Symbol: Music and the External World*, trans. W.R. Trask, Bollingen Series XLIV. Princeton: Princeton University Press.

Chapter 2

Good Looking: Learning to be a Cattle Breeder

Cristina Grasseni

This chapter is based on an ethnographic study of contemporary cattle breeding in northern Italy, both in traditional settings in the mountains and in industrialised settings in the plains. My contribution is based on participant observation among dairy breeders: with breed inspectors, cattle-fair judges and artificial inseminators whose standard practices and expert judgement are integral to the socio-technical system of modern dairy farming. On the one hand, the agribusinesses in the plains boast a deep entrenchment of biotechnology with breeding 'aesthetics', i.e. with the educated capacity of perceiving the animal body in terms of 'functional' beauty. On the other hand, breed selection, especially in marginal rural areas such as the foothills of the Alps, is currently challenged in terms of its ecological sustainability. Hence, to choose between Alpine Brown or Friesian cows ('milk machines', or 'Ferraris', as often commented by alpine breeders with mixed awe and sneering) is felt as a question of personal ethical and aesthetic commitment. Behind the idealised icon of cows grazing on untouched alpine meadows, this ethnographic investigation reveals an ongoing and active negotiation of local, historical and tacit knowledge vis-à-vis standard world-wide technology, repositioning the Alps within the world-wide dynamics of a 'global hierarchy of value' (Herzfeld 2004).

As I have explained elsewhere (Grasseni 2005), the cows that are currently bred in Valtaleggio, the site of my fieldwork, are 'Superbrown' cows, i.e. they are the offspring of heifers of Brown Breed stock that were sired with imported semen of top-ranking American bulls. These, in turn, are the result of a programme of breed selection that started when Swiss Brown specimens were imported from the Swiss Alps to the American Midwest in the 1880s. After the Second World War, selected sires from the American Brown breed were used to 'improve' the local breeds of the alpine valleys. Therefore, the animals that now graze 'Heidi'-type pastures in Lombardy are the result of this double movement of commodities (animals and semen) across the Atlantic Ocean. The impact of 'brownization', nevertheless, is felt both in terms of loss of biodiversity and in terms of loss of 'authenticity', while on the other hand it has been pushed through in the last decades as the recipe for progress and development, for integration in world-wide markets and networks of professional hierarchies and events. This opposition characterises the issue of rural development amongst dairy farmers in the Italian Alps. Whilst the traditional skills of animal husbandry were conveyed through domestic apprenticeship, the application of biotechnology and of mechanisation within current farming practices also entails a redefinition of breeding skills.

Here I hope to show the workings of just one of these all-pervading micro-processes through which new professional identities are shaped. I aim at showing how difficult it is to contest and distance oneself from social meanings, hegemonic aesthetics and moral orders that are created at the level of embodied skills belonging to 'taskscapes'.[1] In particular, I focus here on skilled vision, tacit knowledge and social mimicry as fundamental factors in the formation of professional identities. Specifically, I wish to show how a vast array of devices mediates, shapes and allows the breeders' perception, expression and representation of cows. These devices include: templates for the 'ideal cow'; diagrams of her 'functional traits'; protocols of conduct for cattle fair judges; professional and amateur videos made by breeders at cattle fairs; eloquent and colourful commercial adverts for bull semen; listings of the best bulls, heifers, calves and embryos available on the market – and, tellingly, *toys*. All these are both carriers of international standards and ecological items in one's immediate locality, educating attention and constituting communities of practice. Crucially, the history of 'technical mediation' (Latour 1994) in the world of animal husbandry and the enskilment of the breeder's vision go hand in hand. The aim of this case study is to throw some light on to the following issues: how do aesthetic conventions draw boundaries between different perceptions of 'proper' professional conduct? How are claims of belonging expressed, embodied and performed in local skills? How can critical debates about biodiversity, selection and improvement compete with a hegemonic identity discourse on a common terrain?

In what follows I shall first outline a brief history of the origin of the kind of animal representation that we find embodied in these artefacts. Then I shall present an ethnographic case highlighting the role played by a tacit 'aesthetics' in the formation of a breeder's skilled vision. The case deals with the specific use of toy cows by the children of dairy farmers and of other practitioners associated with cattle breeding. The analysis that follows will highlight the resemblance between toy cows and the templates used by professional breed experts to evaluate dairy cows at cattle fairs and for the national herdbook. This item shows a link between the ecology of the visual environments of the children and that of the expert practitioners that inhabit their adult world of reference.

Histories of Animal Representation and the Designer Cow

The social and technical impact of agri-biotechnology dates back to the Age of Improvement and has since shaped farmers' perception of animal worth. In other words, there exists a direct link between animal representation, agricultural improvement and the ecology of vision of the rural landscape. Even before the inception of photographic records, artists painted their contemporaries in their environment, displaying their wealth: when it came to agricultural innovators, this meant their mansions and the surrounding estates, their horses and carriages, their cattle, sheep and pigs. Up until the end of the eighteenth century, though, the only class that could afford to commission oil paintings would have portraits of their ancestors made for their galleries - the land and animals that guaranteed them their titles of gentility were not the object of their reflexive representation. The great landowners were educated in the sensibility of Arcadia, the bucolic and later the picturesque by the Grand Tour, the collection of classic antiquities and the first development of sight-seeing tourism (Barrell 1980; see also Berger 1972).

But already throughout the eighteenth century, in the increase of the urban population and the Industrial Revolution, lay the conditions, firstly in Britain, for the enclosures and improvement movement, which made the land an object of careful scrutiny, representation and intervention. By the turn of the century, with the import of choice livestock (Dutch cattle, Arabian horses and Siamese pigs), selective inbreeding produced the first thoroughbred breeds, first racehorses, then beef cattle, pigs and sheep. At this point, already well acquainted with the social significance of human portraiture, the members of the landed gentry were eager to have their achievements put on record. By the first half of the nineteenth century animal portraiture became much sought after, while the lesser, or less well established artists produced engravings and mezzotints for those who could not afford oil paintings (Clutton-Brock and Hall 2002). Public taste became acquainted with celebratory portraits of oxen and bulls, of dams and sheep, of their proud owners and their landscaped gardens. This new education of attention established the canon of the ideal type, which we still see at work in contemporary breeding. For instance, there are handbooks and even professional jobs aimed at explaining and applying all the tricks of the trade to make a cow look good, both in terms of toileting the fur, tail and hooves and in terms of putting her in the right posture for a cattle fair exhibition or a magazine cover (see Telfer 1994; Willis 1999; or www.anarb.it). Nowadays the tradition established through this social history of animal portraiture survives – and thrives – not in the form of paintings, but in photographic records, in computer-generated 'models of the ideal cow', and even in plastic toys, as I shall dwell on later. How did this aesthetics come about?

The introduction of selective breeding plays an important part in the political history of 'improvement' - about which recent science-historical theses have stressed the paramount links between the European colonial enterprise and the capacity to develop a network of apt representations of nature.[2] This process involved naturalists, agricultural professionals and the landed gentry. In Britain, the enclosures movement began and took hold in the second half of the eighteenth century, progressively putting an end to the open fields system and to the occupation of the peripheral strips of the states by landless peasants, a practice that dated back to the Middle Ages (Fussell 1984: 13–26).[3] The Agricultural Revolution saw the rise of the new fodder crops: clover, turnips, rye or rye grass, lucern and sainfoin. From 1760, with the patronage of King George III (known as 'Farmer George'), a generation of agricultural pioneers and popularisers (amongst whom was Arthur Young) and a number of institutions and societies were ready to emerge. The Board of Agriculture (1793) of John Sinclair, though short-lived, provided a complete review of the kingdom's farms in the *County Reports*. The more fortunate Royal Agricultural Society of England, the Bath and West of England Society (1777), the Highland Agricultural Society (1784), and especially the Smithfield Club (1798) cultivated overlapping interests with the Society for the Encouragement of Arts and the Royal Society of Arts, Manufacture and Commerce. The latter, founded in 1754, offered prizes for farming experiments as well as stimulating the art of painting and drawing (Fussell 1984: 26–45).

The vast majority of the cattle population, though, remained largely 'all purpose' until nearly the end of the nineteenth century, that is, it was used both for milk and meat, and also put to work as plough and draught oxen. As Ritvo (1987) notices, in fact, the craze for massive animals was part of a nationalist rhetoric favouring the dominant landed gentry, which, fostering class distinction, had relatively little impact on the actual farming production and so was inefficient vis-à-vis the overall rationale of actual improvement. As in the changing social landscape of marginal rural areas in Europe today, we find a distinct clash of interests between the abstract agenda of breed selection which makes use of a hegemonic discourse of 'improvement', and the grounded concerns of professional farmers who try to apply useful information to their immediate surroundings and specific environments (see Grasseni 2005). The development of a standard livestock industry was a slow process that was only first encouraged after the middle of the eighteenth century by the need for red meat for factory workers, and tallow for oiling machines and for lighting. Indeed, it took a whole 'age of improvement' – not only a class of inventive landowners but also a lot of publicity and advertising – to change the course of history, and of nature. Until then, it was mostly up to inventive local squires to experiment with new crops and systems of fertilisation of the light soils (Fussell 1984: 3–13; see also Fussell 1966).[4] But the Age of Improvement, with its shows, pamphlets and propaganda, established the necessary network of gentlemen of science (agricultural experimenters, surveyors and publicists) that made local efforts known and concerted, changing for ever the landscape and livestock patrimony, previously infinitely varied, complex and localised.[5]

The expertise and cross-breeding experiments developed by the aristocrats for racing and hunting horses, which had been developed from a very narrow group of imports, created an important precedent for livestock breeders. The strategy of 'like engendering like' in animal husbandry produced outstanding beef exemplars. Robert Bakewell (1725–95) of Dishley Grange near Loughborough experimented with intensive inbreeding of his best stock, developing the New Leicestershire breed of sheep and the Longhorn breed of cattle. He was followed by the Colling brothers, the improvers of the Teeswater cattle after the import of Dutch Shorthorns. They established a dual purpose (dairy and beef) Shorthorn breed that dominated the British cattle industry until the specialised Friesians (themselves widely crossed with imports of English Shorthorns during the nineteenth century) took over as the prime dairy breed after the Second World War (see Fraser 1972; Stanley 1995; Whitlock 1977).

Crucially, a number of topographical and animal painters were employed to record the results of estate improvement.[6] According to the historian of agriculture G.E. Fussell (1984), it was indeed animal portraiture that developed the sense of the countryside as a pictorial scene in its own right: the Norwich School of East Anglia had already been influenced by the Dutch School, while Thomas Gainsborough (1727–88) and George Stubbs were precursors of the established landscapists of the nineteenth century, Turner and Constable. Previously, the appearance of the English landscape had been worthy of notice in the eyes of the educated elite only if horrific, magnificent or wild, following the lesson of Salvator Rosa, Poussin and Claude. In other words, it was the familiarity with the 'classics', often connected with the Grand Tour prescribed to the sons of the aristocracy, that served as a veritable education of visual taste in a restricted circle.[7] In the last decades of the eighteenth century, then, *picturesque* became the catchword for the genteel elite, following the success of William Gilpin's volumes of description of the national scenery after his tours (1769–1806). Conversely, the fad of landscape gardening began, with extended pieces of estates transformed so that the owner and his guests might enjoy a good view from their strolls among artificial ponds, ha-has and ornamental cottages. This too contributed to a striking metamorphosis of the English landscape: from bog, heath and rough pasture to enclosed clover fields and scenic gardens. Anyone travelling the country – which became more necessary because of the increasing amounts of goods being exchanged and transported – could not have avoided the view of such great changes. The production of a new mode of representing the rural landscape and its human and animal inhabitants was encouraged by the real change in the visible appearance of the landscape brought about by the politics of improvement. From seeking magnificent sights in the Highlands or the Lake District, genteel taste shifted to the delightful scenes of stately homes, flourishing fields and landscaped gardens that were in fact the settings for improved animal husbandry and breeding experiments (for the development of gardens as a medium for the visual integration and domestication of nature into the everyday ecology of the landed gentry, see Browne 1996.)

Animal paintings and prints were the access point for the subaltern landed gentry into an international theory of agricultural improvement, and a site for celebration of those personalities of the aristocracy who exerted their social and political influence towards 'Improvement' (see Ritvo 1987: 6–10). In late eighteenth-century London there was an increasing market of subaltern gentry who could not afford oil paintings but could settle for aquatints and engravings after the originals. The workshop of engraver Raphael Smith and the talent of yet-to-be established painters such as George Morland (1763–1804), and James Ward (1769–1859), catered for this market. Landscape painting differed greatly from the settings of the Agricultural Revolution, as each meant very different outlooks, though some of the early landscapists kept shifting, with some unease, between landscape and animal painting, or the always well-remunerated art of the portrait (Beckett 1993). Animal portraits, especially of cattle, became highly sought after, and many artists obliged: Gainsborough, Ward, Stubbs, but especially Thomas Weaver (1774–1843) and Thomas Bewick (1753–1828). Bewick, in particular, became a renowned cattle expert after the publication of his *General History of*

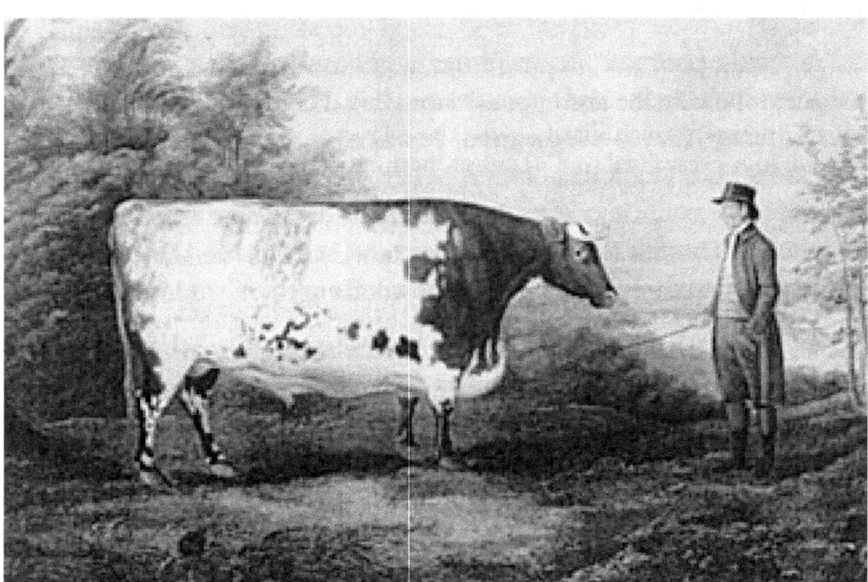

Figure 2.1 *Durham Ox (1802), engraving by I. Whessel after an oil painting by John Boultbee (1753–1812).* (Courtesy of the Museum of English Rural Life, The University of Reading)

Quadrupeds (1790) and painted several outstanding exemplars, until he grew fastidious about owners' requests to fake the pictures. In fact, the first 'improvements' led to celebrating massive, even monstrous exemplars regardless of their reproductive capacity or of the quality of the meat produced: the Collings bred the notorious Durham Ox (1796–1807) (Figure 2.1), 165 centimetres high, weighing 1.3 tons, who was in fact paraded for a fee until his death, in keeping with the contemporary fad for showing exotic or 'freak' animals. Famously portrayed by Thomas Weaver and by John Boultbee (1753–1812) in 1802, it was so popular that 2,000 copies of his portrait were ordered in the first year of shows. After this vogue, portraits of cattle tended to assume conventionally static postures, rather than being drawn in real-life scenes, highlighting the rectangular bulky body of both oxen and bulls, and even adding fat bulges at the cost of verisimilitude (see Quinn 1993; Ritvo 1987: 69–79; Whitlock 1977: 112–21). As Ritvo argues, the pompous and wasteful celebration of simply 'massive' animals was more a rhetorical strategy that re-stated aristocratic dominance and class distinction by strongly connecting it to the issue of pedigree, rather than a genuine striving for utilitarian improvement – a goal that was nevertheless shared by farming entrepreneurs and breeding professionals such as Robert Bakewell (1987: 45–81).

The need for systematic knowledge soon resulted in series of paintings being commissioned – and even scale plaster models – of exemplars of various breeds, since 'neither question – how to distinguish breeds from each other and what standards to apply to individuals of given breeds – had been completely settled by the end of the eighteenth century' (Ritvo 1987: 65).[8] The agricultural shows accompanying the summer season of sheep shearing were important meeting points, events of social celebration, competition and prize-winning. Those held on the estates of Thomas Coke Earl of Leicestershire (at Holkham in Norfolk) and of the Duke of Bedford (at Woburn Abbey) were expensive social events hosting many agricultural celebrities, staging ploughing competitions, and ending in memorable banquets (see Ritvo 1987: 70–71). As is explained below they played a similar social and professional function to contemporary cattle fairs and gatherings of specialised breed associations nowadays. Pictures, paintings, engravings and daguerreotypes served as records of such occasions: the Woburn sheep shearing was immortalised by George Garrard, who portrayed himself in the act of presenting his models of sheep breeds to the Duke's sons.

Since the end of the eighteenth century, animal portraits have carried messages for those who know the background of the animals' fame and worth. To the inexperienced eye, they may look like idiosyncratic depictions of oversized, overfed, overdisplayed freaks. To a specialised community of practice, though, they conveyed a powerful novelty of wealth, social change and confidence in 'advancement'. Animal representation was and is, in a sense, a tool for the education of attention. This is why the social history of animal portraiture can explain some of the roots of our everyday ecology of perception, filtering our capacity to read and understand the shapes and looks of contemporary domestic and industrial animals. The experimentation of the Age of Improvement was soon followed by the specialisation of farming districts and breeds: for instance the Shorthorn dual-type breed split into beef and dairy Shorthorns early in the nineteenth century. The new breed societies, with their herdbooks, registries and codes for the public evaluation of prize animals at institutionalised cattle fairs, ensured that the breeds' distinctive traits were maintained, attended to and handed down. Through selection, and, later, artificial insemination, the 'improved' traits of the peak achievers were thus spread to the rest of the herd.

The spread of a hegemonic aesthetics of breeding was since the beginning a geopolitical process, mixing natural, national and moral economies. For the same reasons for which 'the eighteenth century's most renowned naturalists – Banks, Buffon, Haller, Linnaeus – served as consultants to the Crown in agricultural and medical matters' (Spary 1996: 186), the establishment of a dominant standard 'natural economy' of domestic cattle contributed to the growing imperialism well into the nineteenth century. With colonialism, the British livestock industry provided the cattle herds of Australia, New Zealand, South Africa and the Americas. The tradition of animal portraiture that had been established was therefore instrumental to the globalising strategy of breed improvement. In fact, the genre established in the Age of Improvement is still predominant as a 'breeding aesthetic', and continues to this day, in the form of photographs of posing champion-cows at agricultural exhibitions, livestock catalogues for sale – nowadays available on line – and even video recordings, taken with amateur camcorders at cattle fairs by the farmers themselves (see Grasseni 2004a).

Since the inception of artificial insemination, then, bull progeny testing has become paramount to cattle breeding. Especially in the dairy industry, where the morphology can be closely related to, and become a measure of, potential productivity, the prescribed 'milking traits' have become a canon for longevity and functionality for birth-giving and machine-milking. The traits are evaluated with numerical scores by professional breed experts, both in the shed and at cattle fairs. Such 'morpho-functional evaluations' are combined with the measured milk production to calculate 'genetic indexes', which are aimed to express the desirability of the cow as a reproducer and the strengths of the sire for improving selected traits. The body of the cow is hence 'translated' in numeric scores, listings and classifications that form the basis of cattle marketing. In the case of the dairy industry, a 'linear system of evaluation' for dairy cows was introduced in the USA at the end of the 1980s, consisting of nineteen templates that indicate which is the best shape for relevant traits of the dairy cow's body. Each trait is both described and represented visually. A numerical score is associated with a range of proximity to the prescribed shape, by comparison with the less favourable form that the same trait might take on (see Figure 2.2). The recommended shape that the trait in question should have (for instance, dorsal line, udder depth, or teats direction) is highlighted in a box, by comparison with less recommendable configurations of the back, udder or limbs. With the introduction of this system, qualitative judgements such as 'outstanding', 'acceptable' or 'mediocre', were replaced with marks from 1 to 50: a measure of perfection, or rather of distance from perfection. If breed experts used meter and scale (which they don't, but only for 'practical and economic difficulties'), the result would be an objective and repeatable *biological measure* of the animal. This strategy to 'translate' aesthetic judgement into numerical statements is a deliberate move towards standardisation, working within the logic of 'translatability' and 'accountability' that makes globalisation and commodification so successful (see Grasseni 2005).

This strategy, however, is politically controversial and highly ideological, since it takes no consideration of issues such as the loss of biodiversity, the environmental unsustainability of intensive breeding and the optimal adaptation of local, 'unimproved' breeds to specific terrains and climates – as is becoming evident with the world-wide effects of agribusiness. In the light of this, and paradoxically, while there is increasing interest, amongst specialist circles, for the reintroduction of local, diversified breeds – thus striving to erase the effects of two hundred years of standardisation – the aesthetics of breed selection has become hegemonic even at the level of common sense. Contemporary animal aesthetics is so pervaded by token prototypes of excellence that our average perception of cattle approximates the form of the 'ideal cow'. The rift with the 'natural' characteristics of local breeds is such that only zoological connoisseurs could name more than a handful of breeds, and many original stocks have become extinct. Nevertheless, the ecology of everyday perception within the community of practitioners that deal with the livestock industry is forcefully shaped by semen adverts (Figure 2.3), videos and posters of cattle fair winners, and models of ideal types (Figure 2.4), which, as we shall see next, even take the form of plastic toy-cows for children to play with (Figure 2.5).

The Role of Artefacts in Professional Aesthetics

A long iconographic history and a pragmatically minded practice of portraiture, exhibition and scrutiny of the animal body both inform and shape the current perception of animal nature, especially amongst communities of experts, as documented in the breeding contexts of display (such as cattle fairs) and distribution (such as professional publications, magazines, web sites). I now wish to analyse ethnographically contemporary materials, showing how *small mediators* can be enormously relevant and instrumental to the make-up of the 'continuous worlds' (Ingold 1993) that we move in as taskscapes. I do so by looking at the practical seamlessness of experience, though noticing also that everyday practicalities are sedimentations of historical, political and economic processes. In particular, I

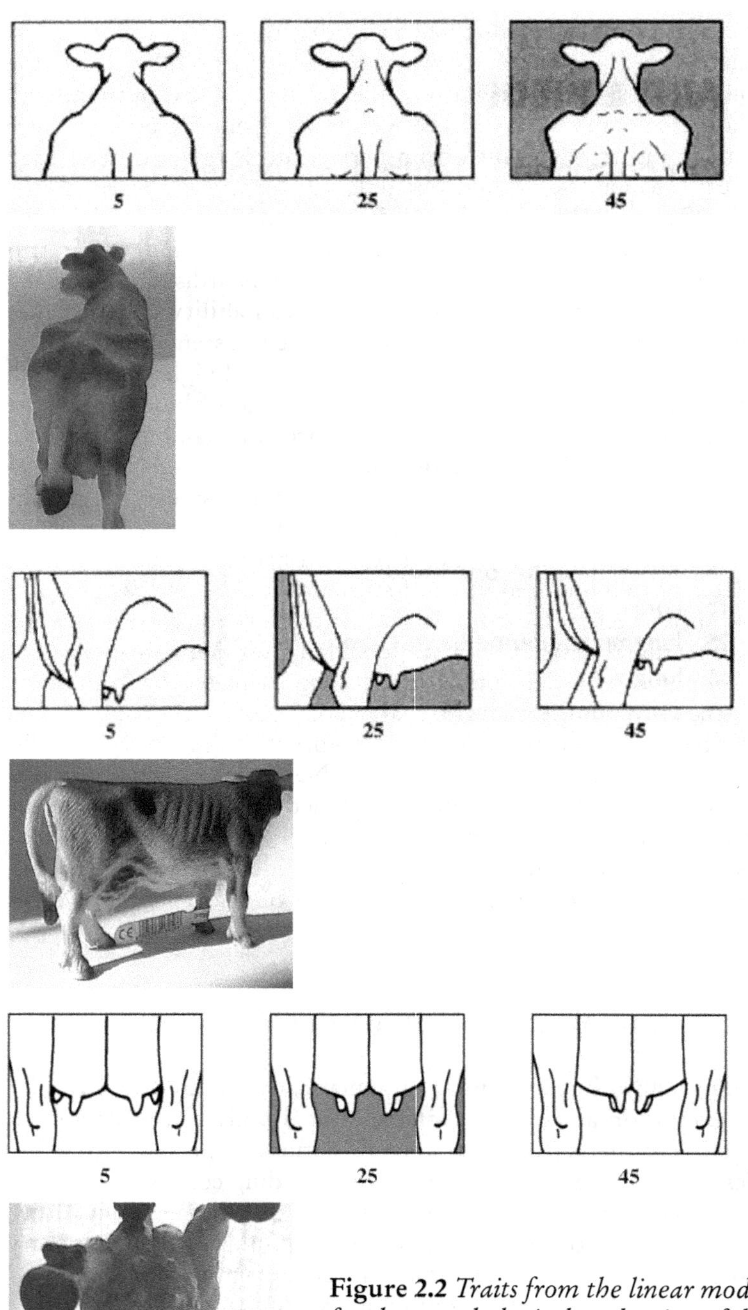

Figure 2.2 *Traits from the linear model for the morphological evaluation of dairy cows (courtesy of A.N.A.R.B.) compared with relevant traits of a plastic toy cow.* (Photos: C. Grasseni)

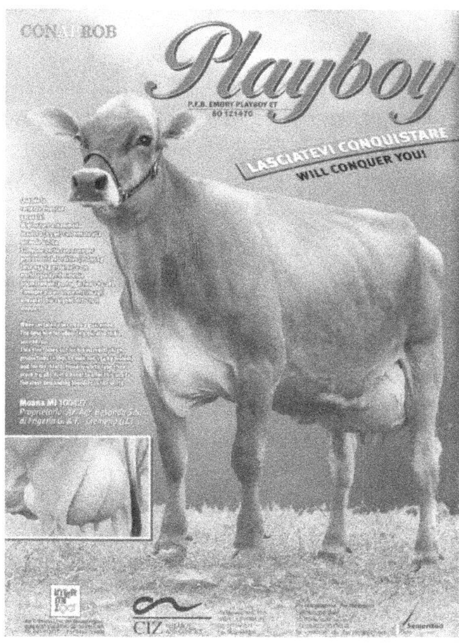

Figure 2.3 *Semen advert for the bull 'Playboy',* Razza Bruna *38(6): 8 (November 1998).* (Courtesy of A.N.A.R.B.)

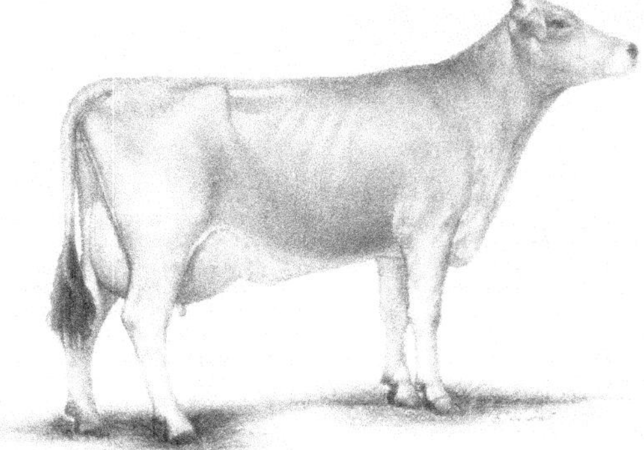

Figure 2.4 *Model of the ideal Italian cow of the Brown breed.* (Courtesy of A.N.A.R.B.)

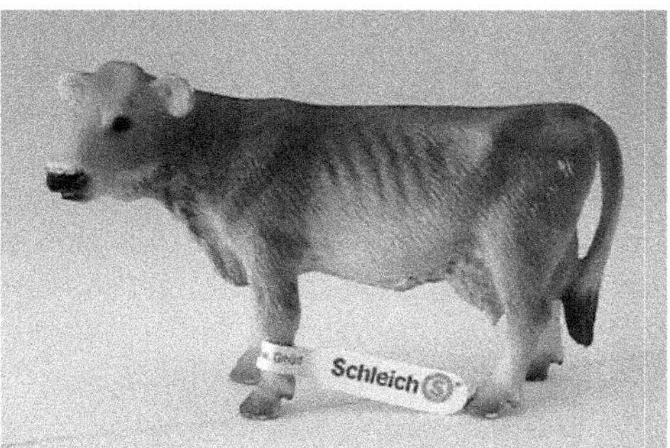

Figure 2.5 *Plastic toy cow made in China for Schleich, Germany, 2001.* (Photo: C. Grasseni)

try to pinpoint some of those small mediators in artefacts, meant in a Latourian way as *actants* in a network (Latour 1994).

To start with, let me then introduce ethnographically some children, and their parents, whom I met during my ethnographic fieldwork in alpine Lombardy, at the foot of the Italian Alps. Patrizio is an agricultural adviser, a technician with a degree in agricultural sciences who served his apprenticeship in the cadres of the farmers' union, in the valleys north of Bergamo. His work consisted in visiting farmers, helping them update their herdbook, informing them about aid and funding opportunities for improvements to their herd or stable, filling out forms for them when these contain too many technicalities, submitting proposals on their behalf and informing them when funding has been approved. He also visited cheese-making facilities, advising on the process of curdling the milk, on how to best season the fresh cheese, and alerting the producers to the best opportunities for advertising and selling their products. The high-quality cheeses produced in the mountains sell at local fairs, or through the cooperative network, or at bigger events held at Bergamo's Fair pavilion. They also sell further away – for instance, at the many events organised by Milan's Chamber of Commerce, or by the Slow Food Association, which strives to preserve organic and traditional foods, or again by the Association for Breeders of the Alpine Brown, who are lobbying for the construction of a niche market for cheese that is made entirely out of Brown cows' milk. Patrizio himself does not come from a farming background, though he was born in a small village in the low mountains at the mouth of Val Brembana, half-an-hour's drive from Bergamo, at the foot of the Lombard Alps. He grew up collecting wood on his property that stretched back on a steep slope behind the stone house, chatting with the elderly who still kept the occasional goat or sheep to graze their land. His relatives fatten a pig for slaughtering in winter, and he receives his share of salami within a network of friends and kin. He prepared his university exams in the glow of a wood-burning stove. As a graduate working for the farmers' union, a political engagement in the local administration was almost natural for him. Elected to the town council and to the town local government board, he was then chosen by the Mayor as referent for agriculture. He was then nominated for the whole of Val Brembana's Mountain Community council, and selected by its President as *Assessore* for agriculture (namely, the member of the Mountain Community organ of local government who is in charge of agricultural matters).

I visited him and his family over Christmas 2004, and I met his little son of three, Emilio. Patrizio had taken him to visit the farm of some of his closest customers, farmers with whom trust and esteem usually combine to create reliable, and sometimes durable, political allegiances. Emilio owns a collection of plastic toy cows, which he proceeded to 'milk' as a gift-performance for me. At his father's prompting, he first pretended to wash his hands, then sanitised the cow's teats, then imitated with his mouth the sound of milk flowing from the teats, while with his clumsy little hands he mimicked the alternating movements of the sucking cylinders of a milking machine. Of course, no one milks by hand any more, perhaps some remote pensioner who still has a couple of old cattle, and an *Assessore* would not visit the modest owner of two cows over Christmas. No, the farmer they visited had a milking parlour, and Emilio had been exposed to the protocols of self-management that all farms enforce as a legal requirement – HACCP or Hazard Analysis Critical Control Point.[10] Emilio's ecology of everyday practice, at the age of three, is forcefully shaped by his father's activity, and consequently by international protocols of 'good practice' in standard agribusiness.

Similarly, in my previous fieldwork in a nearby valley (1997–99), I witnessed the mimetic games of children of Brown breed farmers, using plastic toy cows. While I was living with a family of dairy farmers, I observed my host's son playing with toy cows on the pastures. When I video-recorded his games, Marco was ten years old and was playing with his best friend, the son of the local mountain refuge-keeper. They were intent on a complex exercise of social mimicry: pretending to be responsible and well-advised herders. Marco and his playmate had found a natural hollow slope in the terrain, probably caused by a small landslide after the spring rains, and had carved out from the bare soil what looked like a miniature mountain pasture. They had carved a wide road for their various toy trucks and used the steeper path only for their toy motorbikes. They showed me their development plans:

J. – Here we can come up with the truck and load goats, pigs, chickens, everything ...
M. – We have fenced that side off with electric wire so they don't stray off.
J. – We have built this road for the motorbikes ...
M. – ... or also for the cows.
J. – Yes, then there's the big road, for the truck. It's big enough so if there's two at once, one coming up and one coming down, they can both fit.

They had horses, chickens and sheep laid out. But the cows had a separate space, grazing peacefully, well scattered on a plain, and well protected by a fence. Marco was pointing out to me which animals belonged to whom (whether to himself or to his friend), and how they were related between themselves. Identifying the animals by the relations between them (mother of, father of, sisters, twins, etc.) also meant identifying which toy belonged to whom. About the horses:

M. – Five are mine, also this Dad and Mum are mine. All the others belong to Jacopo.
J. – I got four new horses at Christmas, then also the cows lying on their side and these two bulls.

About the bulls, which were kept separated in a fence by the side of the pasture:

M.- These two are mine. This cow is the mother of this bull, this one is the mother of that one, these two belong to Jacopo, and this one is the mother of that.

About the cows:

M. – These are my Brown twins. Then there are three sisters here and that one is their Mum.
I – How many are there altogether?
M. – We did not count them. Er …
J. – Let's see … 31. No, 32 …
M. – There's one taking water at the spring. It's Jacopo's. There's also her calf. All of the cows lying on the side belong to Jacopo. Plus the one standing by the bull ranch.
J. – Those with a piece of rubber belong to Marco.
M. – Plus that one who lost the rubber ring …

Marco was reproducing the discerning knowledge that breeders have of their cattle, as well as their keen sense of property. He applied to his toys the skilled vision that his father applied to real cows. In fact, he was exercising that skill every day on the real animals as well, distinguishing between them and calling them by their names, learning their genealogies and noticing the similarities and differences amongst them (see Grasseni 2004b). While he was displaying his expertise in his miniature world, it was of importance to him to remark that 'When I was not even two years old, one day there was a cattle fair at the cooperative and we exhibited our best cows. The others showed their best cows as well. I was not even two, but I led a cow in the ring'.

In other words, Marco was engaging from very early on in what Jean Lave calls 'legitimate peripheral participation' (Lave and Wenger 1991) in a community of practice – and was proudly aware of it. Learning to be a breeder implies an education of attention that starts at an early age, a veritable apprenticeship in skilled vision (Grasseni 2004b). It may be unsurprising that exercises in social mimicry may be replicas of adult worlds that are played out in secrecy and in a separate, self-made space. But if compared with children's games of the 'traditional past', what strikes one is the specialisation, both of the artefact and of the accompanying gaze. Toys in the past, as noticed by alpine anthropologists, ethnologists, folklore specialists and experts of material culture, were functional for an immediate introduction to the activities of adult life, and could be hand-made within the family, either by the children themselves as prototypes of more skilled artefacts, or directly borrowed from the tools and objects of everyday activities (Angioni 1984). Here we have purpose-made, design toys that resemble the shape of purpose-bred, design cows. The fact is, in other words, that even plastic toy cows reproduce the ideals of good form that are to be found in cattle fairs' champions and models. By manipulating them daily the breeders' children incorporate the hegemony of agribusiness and of 'improved' aesthetics into their everyday ecology of attention.

I realised this when I myself started 'playing' breeder with a toy cow, trying to assess its traits using the 'linear module for the evaluation of traits' (Figure 2.2 above) that is recommended by the National Association of Brown Breeders, currently used in cattle fairs for ranking specimens of the Brown breed. I compared the nineteen traits of the linear module with the corresponding parts of the toy's body, pairing up the graphs representing the recommended look of each trait and purpose-made photographs of the toy that I took from different angles. I then realised that the toy's shape had been modelled on the basis of the same traits by which the dairy cow's body can be broken down into the 'linear model'. In fact, the toy cow is not simply compatible with a functional evaluation model, but it actually reproduces a miniature version of the model cow of the Association of the Brown Breed breeders (see Figure 2.4 above). In other words, the toy's shape mimics the ideal of good form that is found in cattle fair champions, boasting for instance a mighty udder. There are, nevertheless, a number of shortcomings, probably due to the needs of machine-casting and pressing, such as a certain coarseness of the limbs that contributes to an overall impression of a rather squat and sturdy animal – far from the lean and fine shapes of cattle fair champions. To this degree of detail, miniaturisation does not seem to work. But the fundamental factors of breed selection have been taken on: for instance, the toy cow has a straight top line, which is a sign of strength and vigour and facilitates birth-giving in a real animal. The visible ribs testify angularity – or dairy form – a sign of the 'productive potential' of milking cows. In fact, a hyperthyroideic metabolism 'burns' excess fat and yields extra milk. The udder shows swollen lactiferous veins, and symmetrically placed teats, ideal for machine-milking. The computer-generated 'model of the ideal Italian cow of the Brown Breed' in fact is close enough, especially in its most apparent features (straight back, udder size, teats placement, udder veins, hyperthyroid metabolism resulting in lean bones, etc.). In this sense, the toy is a prime example of standardisation, while it acts itself as a model of standardised animals.

To put it briefly, this toy has a function that depends on its shape and on its looks. Conversely, we can compare this toy with any type of animal-shaped cuddly toy. Their appeal lies in the material, in the texture that affords softness and invites manipulation, but their function is exhausted in the immediacy of their soothing action. The plastic toy cow instead allows the detachment and the discernment of vision – a theme on which Rane Willerslev elaborates in the previous chapter. Because of that, this artefact carries technical knowledge and aesthetic sensibility into the ecology of practice of the children who manipulate it daily in their games. But not only that. It's a whole world and its history – a form of life: social *and* cognitive, political *and* ecological – that is tangled up in a toy. The toy synthesises the expert knowledge of the community of practice of the breeders of the Brown breed. These are farmers who invest in breed selection and programme the inseminations of their cattle, choosing which traits should be enhanced in order to increase the animals' potentials for production. The toy thus embodies an aesthetic and functional ideal that has been shaped and handed down in the history of animal husbandry since the inception of animal portraiture in conjunction with the Age of Improvement (discussed above). It also confirms the demise and marginalisation of traditional breeding and the hegemonic success of standard forms (both in toys and in animals) despite recent attempts at re-implementing the biodiversity of local alpine breeds, in conjunction with the rediscovery of typical products and organic foods. For instance, the toy has no horns. It is not a 'natural'-looking animal at all, but rather the result of standard interventions that are typical of modern dairy farming – such as burning the horns at the roots, to avoid risks of clashes between the animals, and to orient the whole body to the sole function of milk production. By its very shape this toy testifies to how established and pervasive is the aesthetics associated with the standardisation of animal husbandry.

The toy, like a cattle fair champion, looks *beautiful* and *proper* to a trained eye. For this very reason, it reminds us that hegemony may well inhabit, and be reinforced by, beautiful simplicity, or 'simply' beauty. In other words, there is a very complex simplicity at work in what is perceived synthetically as 'grace'. What part is the toy cow going to play in the child's life? And where would it derive its alleged power to influence, guide and shape his skilled vision, his convictions about what is a beautiful cow, what is a good breeding practice, and what is a breeding achievement? In order to answer, one needs to look a bit higher. To be precise, one needs to look up to his father's kitchen cupboard. (Figure 2.6)

In October 2004 I revisited the cattle fair of the valley where I carried out fieldwork between 1997 and 2000. Marco's family won virtually all the prizes, having established themselves as the champions of Brown breed selection and of 'modernisation' in the valley. I was invited for lunch, and it struck me that there were some model cows sitting on top of the kitchen cupboard. Agapito, Marco's father and a Brown breed expert belonging to the National Association, proudly explained: 'in order to understand how to better a cow you have to be able to detect her faults by comparison with an ideal model. The model is that one', he said, pointing to the top of the cupboard. The cow models on display there were not toys, but trophies won at cattle fairs. There are other types of trophies as well – silver cups, ornamental cow bells, certificates etc. In the summer of 1998 I had helped Marco's grandmother to clean up the garage and we threw away all the garbage – including all the old cups and trophies. We threw away all the silver-plated cups, jumbled them all in the back of the car and took them to the tip. But the model cows were standing even back then, on top of the kitchen cupboard, near the television. These type of model trophies serve a completely different function than the ornamental cups and bells. They embody the expertise that is being

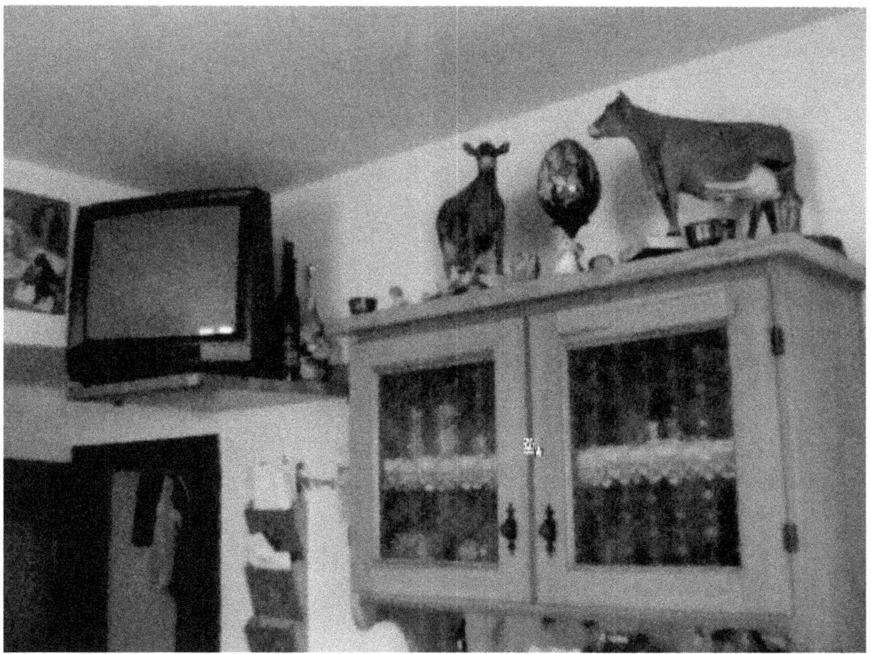

Figure 2.6 *Trophies of cattle fairs in my hosts' kitchen.* (Photo: C. Grasseni)

acknowledged to the breeders who win the prize. They maintain the pedagogical intent and function of the exhibitions held during the Age of Improvement (and of the scale plaster models that were then being cast for the first time), in that they restate the validity of the ideal form that the breeders have purportedly infused in the live flesh of their cows. Their superiority to all other types of trophies was testified by the fact that they were kept well in view, not stored away in a cabinet, nor displayed in the more aseptic context of the farm's office (where all the most recent trophies are displayed), but at the heart of family life – the kitchen, next to the TV.

Conclusion

The ways we see beauty, that we embody skill and enjoy participating in moral order are linked to an ecology of practice. This does not happen solely as a result of the individual workings of the mind, or of the brain, or of the body of each of us, but rather happens through highly socialised means. In particular, I have tried to show ethnographically how the role of specific visual artefacts (with their historical, hegemonic and conflicting sedimentations) is paramount in bridging the gap between the workings of individual minds and macroscopic cultural analysis and critique. The context of learning appears both as a process of growth and an opening up to experience, in all its prosaic, pragmatic and functional character. Children reproduce scale models of the adult activities and relationships that surround them. The skilled vision of breed experts, farmers' children and agricultural advisers is both synthetic and capable of discernment and distinction. I extracted one scale-modelled artefact from the miniature playworld of my hosts' children in order to highlight the pervasive ways in which observational skills and aesthetics are learnt and applied, and how standardisation can work upon this very process. Marco's toy cows are going to play an important role, like the bigger 'model cows' that his father parades in the kitchen and of which he is very proud. And the reason why they are going to play the same function is that they *look* the same. Paradoxically, it is a hegemonic vision, emerging out of learning processes, that maintains their qualities of social, affective and cognitive engagement, of sensuousness, and of creativity.

Notes

1 I refer to the term with which Ingold combines the notions of 'movement through landscape' and 'skilled practice' to render the image of a 'taskscape' as a field in which skilled practitioners learn to 'make their way' (Ingold 1993: 221).

2 In particular see Miller and Reill (1996) and Drayton (2000) on the role of the 'Banksian empire' (Joseph Banks was director of Kew Gardens in London from 1783 till his death in 1829) in the project of a scientific management of world-wide colonial natural resources towards the 'Improvement' of the British Empire.

3 Studying analogous processes of agricultural improvement in Continental Europe, Orland (2003) stresses the link between treating soil, animal and fodder as an economic and ecological unit (starting from the end of the eighteenth century) and the consequent stress on the production of competitive dairy cattle in the nineteenth and twentieth centuries.

4 One of such, Jethro Tull, had designed the first practical seed drill late in the seventeenth century, followed by the invention of threshing machines, chaff cutters and rolling carts.

5 The new expertise drew mostly from the Flemish husbandry and the crop rotation system of the Low Countries – internationally renowned for their gardening techniques - and already observed and reported at the beginning of the seventeenth century.

6 For instance George Stubbs (1724–1806), painter of the renowned Lincolnshire Ox oil painting (1791), commissioned on recommendation by the powerful President of the Royal Society, Sir Joseph Banks, became famous as a horse portraitist, while also painting realist pictures of rural occupations in conjunction with pictures of racehorses in their environment and scenery (Clutton-Brock and Hall 2002: 41).

7 The Dutch masters represented a counter-altar inspired by the more domestic side of life: Rubens (1577–1640), Rembrandt (1606–69), and especially the rural scenes of Paul Potter and Aelbert Cuyp, depicting animals in domestic settings, the field and the barn – even though in these scenes the country itself plays an overwhelming role, with people and animals often featuring as small and insignificant.

8 One of the first attempts by James Ward, commissioned by the Board of Agriculture, remained unpublished due to the bankruptcy of the printer Josiah Boydell (1719–1804) (Beckett 1993: 35–40). George Garrard (1760–1826) completed and published a series of scale plaster models (two-and-a-quarter inches to the foot) under the patronage of the Duke of Bedford, first president of the Smithfield Club in 1800 (Clutton-Brock and Hall 2002: 42).

9 So goes a statement that can be found in Italian on the relevant page of the web site of the National Association of Brown Breed Breeders, www.anarb.it, explaining the methods and principles of morpho-functional evaluations.

10 HACCP was a by-product of the NASA space programme for food supply to manned space flights, aiming to improve health safety by preventing the spoiling of perishable products. Instead of relying on testing finished products, HACCP assesses the risk of occurrence of specific hazards, and controls them at specific stages throughout the entire production process. See Grasseni (2003); Pearson and Dutson (1995).

References

Angioni, G. 1984. 'Tecnica e sapere tecnico nel lavoro preindustriale', *La Ricerca Folklorica* 9: 61–69.

Barrell, J. 1980. *The Dark Side of the Landscape: the Rural Poor in English Painting*, 1730–1840. Cambridge: Cambridge University Press.

Beckett, O. 1993. *The Life and Work of James Ward, 1769–1859. The Forgotten Genius.* Sussex, England: The Book Guild.

Berger, J. 1972. *Ways of Seeing*. London: British Broadcasting Corporation.

Browne, J. 1996. 'Botany in the Boudoir and Garden: the Banksian Context', in *Visions of Empire. Voyages, Botany, and Representations of Nature*, eds. D.P. Miller and P.H. Reill. Cambridge: Cambridge University Press, 153–172.

Clutton-Brock, J. and S.J.G. Hall, 2002. 'All is Useless that Is Not Beef: Stocking the Landscape' in *Love, Labour and Loss: 300 Years of British Livestock Farming in Art*, eds. C. Adams and M. Liversidge (Catalogue). Carlisle: Tullie House Museum and Art Gallery.

Drayton, R. 2000. *Nature's Government: Science, Imperial Britain, and the 'Improvement' of the World.* New Haven: Yale University Press.

Fraser, A. 1972. *The Bull.* Reading: Osprey.

Fussell, G.E. 1966. *The English Dairy Farmer, 1500–1900.* London: Frank Cass & Co.

—— 1984. *Landscape Painting and the Agricultural Revolution.* London: Pindar Press.

Grasseni, C. 2003. 'Packaging Skills: Calibrating Italian Cheese to the Global Market', in *Commodifying Everything: Consumption and Capitalist Enterprise*, ed. S. Strasser. New York: Taylor and Francis, 259–88.

—— 2004a. 'Video and Ethnographic Knowledge: Skilled Vision in the Practice of Breeding', in *Working Images*, eds. S. Pink, A.I. Alfonso and L. Kurti. London: Routledge, 15–30.

—— 2004b. 'Skilled Vision. An Apprenticeship in Breeding Aesthetics', *Social Anthropology* 12 (1): 1–15.

—— 2005. 'Designer Cows: the Practice of Cattle Breeding between Skill and Standardization', *Society and Animals* 13 (1): 33–49. (Online at www.psyeta.org).

Herzfeld, M. 2004. *The Body Impolitic: Artisans and Artifice in the Global Hierarchy of Value.* Chicago: Chicago University Press.

Ingold, T. 1993. 'The Art of Translation in a Continuous World', in *Beyond Boundaries. Understanding, Translation and Anthropological Discourse*, ed. G. Pálsson. London: Berg, 210–30.

Latour, L. 1994. 'On Technical Mediation. Philosophy, Sociology, Genealogy', *Common Knowledge* 3 (2): 29–64.

Lave, J. and E. Wenger 1991. *Situated Learning. Legitimate Peripheral Participation*. Cambridge: Cambridge University Press.

Miller, D.P. and P.H. Reill, eds., 1996. *Visions of Empire: Voyages, Botany, and Representations of Nature*. Cambridge: Cambridge University Press.

Orland, B. 2003. 'Turbo-Cows. About the Production of a Competitive Animal in 19th and early 20th century', in *Industrializing Organisms*, eds. S. Schrepfer and P. Scranton. Piscataway, NJ: Rutgers University Press, 167–90.

Pearson, A.M. and T.R. Dutson, eds. 1995. *HACCP in Meat, Poultry and Fish Processing*. Glasgow: Blackie Academic and Professional.

Quinn, M.S. 1993. 'Corpulent Cattle and Milk Machines. Nature, Art and the Ideal Type', *Society and Animals* 1 (2). (Online at www.psyeta.org).

Ritvo, H. 1987. *The Animal Estate*. Cambridge, Mass.: Harvard University Press.

Spary, E. 1996. 'Political, Natural and Bodily Economies', in *Cultures of Natural History*, eds. N. Jardine, J. Secord and E. Spary. Cambridge: Cambridge University Press, 178–96.

Stanley, P. 1995. *Robert Bakewell and the Longhorn Breed of Cattle*. Ipswich: Farming Press.

Telfer, B. 1994. *Showing Dairy Cattle*. Ipswich: Farming Press.

Whitlock, R. 1977. *Bulls through the Ages*. London: Lutterworth Press.

Willis, M. B. 1999. *Dalton's Introduction to Practical Animal Breeding*. London: Blackwell.

Chapter 3

Icons and Transvestites: Notes on Irony, Cognition and Visual Skill

Francesco Ronzon

> Camp is in the eye of the beholder.
> E. Newton, *Mother Camp*

> I'm a sweet transvestite, from Transsexual, Transylvania.
> *The Rocky Horror Picture Show*

Introduction

Field notes: Verona, Italy; 3/4/ 2003, around midnight, Art Discothèque:

> The man is tall, heavy and muscular. He is dressed in a long evening gown of black satin. The large décolleté reveals a shaved body. The look is refined by heavy make-up, a blonde wig and a flaming red lipstick. The eyes of the audience follow his movements on the stage. His walk is a little trembling because of the high-heeled shoes. Some people shout. Others laugh. When he arrives at centre stage, he starts singing an old pop melody with a wide smile, a loud falsetto and a heavy theatrical pronunciation. In the meantime his hands move in the air tracing lines of shadows in the web of brightly coloured spotlights that surround his figure …

The drag queen show is a typical institution of the gay club and party world of the twentieth and twenty-first centuries. It consists of a rich, ludicrous and flamboyant performance of men acting and dressing like women and implies a peculiar taste for the visual nuances at the roots of mimicking and defacing of gender décor.

In this paper I will make reference to ethnographic materials from fieldwork on the gay world of Verona (Veneto region, northeast Italy), carried out between 2002 and 2004, to investigate how the visual skills of a group of drag queens performing in the area are learned and applied within a situated context.[1] In particular, I will analyse the visual skills of my subjects from an ecological perspective. In the last twenty years, in contrast with the so-called representationalist paradigm,[2] a wide and growing number of researchers in cognitive anthropology have oriented their research emphasising the link between body, world and action (Ingold 2000; Toren 1993; Whitehouse 1996; see Grasseni and Ronzon 2004 for an overview). In this perspective, the eye is not to be considered an organ that elaborates in an inferential way a world of chaotic atomistic sense-data in order to build an internal representation of external reality. On the contrary, eyes are to be considered as part of a wider system of direct perception aimed at picking up the invariants offered by the optical array (the light reflected by the various surfaces of a certain environment) through an active process of research linked to the actions, interests and exploration of the percipient (Gibson 1979).[3] From this hypothesis certain implications follow.

First, vision is a mode of action rather than a prerequisite for action. It is an active and exploratory process of information pick-up; far from working on sensations already received, it involves the continual movement, adjustment and reorientation of the receptor organs themselves.

Second, if vision is a mode of action, then what we 'see' is a direct function of how we act. Depending on the kind of activity in which we are engaged, we will be attuned to picking up particular kinds of information.

Third, within the biological constraints there are no limits to what can be perceived. Throughout life an agent can keep on seeing new 'things' in an otherwise permanent world by a 'fine-tuning' of his visual system to new kinds of information (and this is available to anyone attuned to pick it up).

Finally, and following from the above, one learns to 'see' in the manner appropriate to a culture, not by acquiring programmes or conceptual schemata for organising atomistic sensory data into high-order representation, but by 'hands on' training in everyday tasks whose successful fulfilment requires a practised ability to notice and to respond fluently to salient aspects of the environment. As such, every way of seeing is inseparable from an explicit or implicit 'education of attention' (Gibson 1979: 254). Social agents can not only directly perceive the clues offered by their environments, but also share them. Attuned through prior training and experience to attending to similar invariants, and moving in the same environment in the pursuit of joint activities, they will pick up the same information (Reed 1988: 119–20).

Obviously, this kind of inquiry is not without links and relevance for the cultural anthropological enterprise as a whole. In a certain way, one of the aims of this essay is to persuade the reader that it is only in this ecological perspective that it becomes possible to explain human cognition not only in terms of its neurobiological roots, private mental states or abstract linguistic structure, but also to open up these 'inner' worlds to the history, the culture and the social life of real people acting-in-the world.

Setting

Drag queens are males operating as female impersonators in public performances. Even if they are usually homosexual, they choose to operate as drag queens not from an inner gender compulsion but for artistic and economic purposes. This means that they are artists and do not consider themselves to be female (nor do they want in any way to become women).[4]

Like other Italian drag queens, the troupe of drag queens I studied is part of a marginal and stigmatised[5] 'art world' (Becker 1982). An art world consists of 'all the people whose activities are necessary to the production of the characteristic works which that world defines as art. Members of an art world coordinate the activities by which work is produced by referring to a body of conventional understandings embodied in common practice and in frequently used artifacts' (ibid. 34).[6]

As part of a specific art world, drag queens cooperate repeatedly, even routinely, in similar ways to produce similar works, so that we can think of their art world as an established network of cooperative links among participants. If the same people do not actually act together in every instance, their replacements are also familiar with and proficient in the use of those conventions, so that cooperation can proceed without difficulty. To illustrate the main feature of this art world in the rest of this section I shall offer some information on its origins, social logics and cultural values.

Madame Sisi and His Colleagues

The troupe of drag queens at the centre of this research consists of a team of five to eight members of various ages (from twenty to forty). Even though the troupe experiences a certain turnover, its members generally have a good educational level and come from the Italian middle class (but with no one from the upper strata). In large part, they work in Verona, a rich and large provincial city of northeast Italy. Although the city is located in a very Catholic region (the famous 'Veneto bianco', white Veneto) the local gay world offers various and tolerated low-profile places and activities. The troupe is led by the oldest member of the group (age forty-one), Carlo – or, in art, Madame Sisi[7] (Figure 3.1). He is not only the most expert of the équipe but he is also the owner of Art, a large discothèque where most of the troupe's performances take place.[8] It is a large modern building located in the outskirts of Desenzano (Verona), a little town near Lake Garda (a well-known Italian tourist site). The disco is not targeted exclusively at a gay audience but is notorious for its mixed public (heterosexual and homosexual) and for its exotic, bizarre and transgressive events.[9]

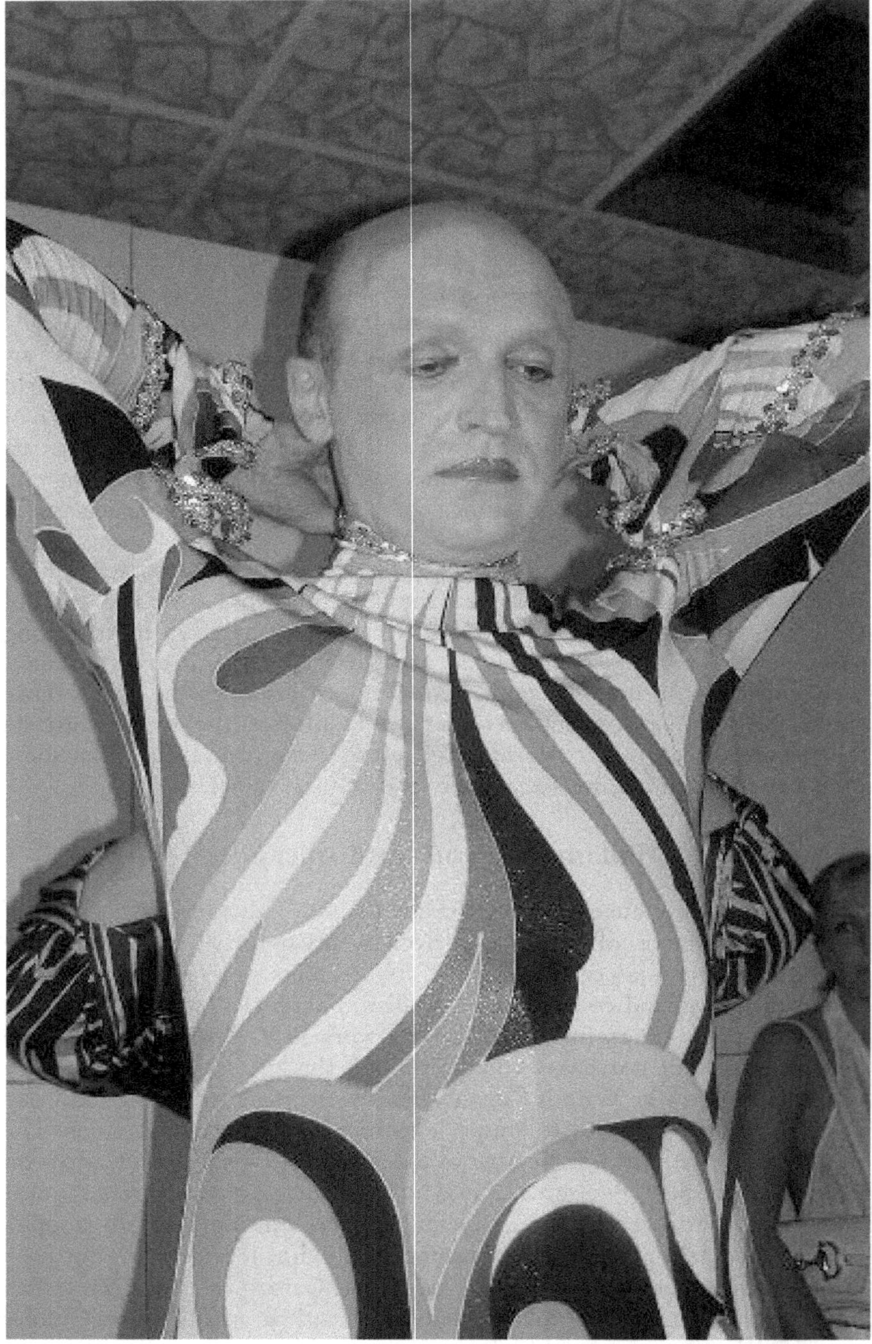

Figure 3.1 *Backstage: Carlo dressing up as Madame Sisi.* (Photo: F. Ronzon)

The artistic numbers performed by my troupe of drag queens include dance, music and dramatic acts. As usual in this art world, the various performances require a combination of beauty and talent (which also determines the pay scale, job hierarchy and social relations of my interlocutors). Quite apart from the specific media, forms and contents of the performances, all of them centre around a logic of *camp*, the core of the drag queen's art. With this expression, drag queens refer in a loose way to any sort of ironic mimicry of gender identity.[10] This effect is achieved by means of two theatrical strategies: first, intentional excess, grotesque and transgression; second, the use of gender code-switching as a marked choice (the alternation between two canons or two varieties of the same gender identity standard). In other words, the logic of camp lies in the tension between maintaining the female personification as closely as possible and breaking it completely so as to force the audience to realise that the imitation is being done by a man. A skilled performer such as Madame Sisi, for example, can create the illusion, break it and pick it up again several time during one song, and the effect can be extremely dramatic and often comic. In other words, to give an effective camp impression demands a highly refined sense of 'look', a sharp sense of timing and, needless to say, a highly developed mimicry skill.

A Brief History of Drag Performance

In order to understand the logic of the art world sustained by Madame Sisi and his colleagues, it is useful to spend some time looking at its origins, evolution and diffusion. In his portrait of gay life in New York up to 1940, George Chauncey devotes much attention to the creation and appropriation of spaces in which gay men were free to be themselves, discussing the gay enclaves in Greenwich Village and Harlem, both of which became tourist attractions, during the pansy 'craze' and the Harlem Renaissance (Chauncey 1994). The most notorious of these appropriated spaces were the Drag Balls.

Starting at the end of the nineteenth century as a gay improvisation on the canon of straight masquerade balls, by the mid-1920s they were attracting thousands of observers and participants (a large percentage of those who attended the Balls were heterosexual, there to observe rather than participate). The drag queens on display at the Balls embodied camp culture in their inversion of gender conventions. The highlight of the Balls was the beauty contest or 'parade of the pansies', in which the fashionably dressed drags would vie for the title of Queen of the Ball. In this way the Balls were a particular source of pride for the fairies and drag queens who were ordinarily derided by 'normals' and 'normal-like' gay men alike.[11] With the advent of legislation and the after-effects of the Depression, the Drag Balls ceased to be such a major event in the eyes of the public. However, gay men have continued to hold Drag Balls and to use drag queen as a means of expression right up to the present day.

As well documented by Esther Newton in the first extensive ethnographic research on the topic (Newton 1972), if in the beginning the Drag Balls were an extension of the effeminate stereotypes used in the initial process of gay self-identification, in the course of time they have become an art performance within the leisure places of both the straight circuits and the homosexual subculture (pub, disco, happening, and so on), to celebrate ordinary holidays and important events in the gay calendar (such as Hallowe'en). This parodying of gender was then taken to its logical extremes by the radical drag queens of the 1970s, who wore drags as a political statement intended to confront or 'freak out' the straight community by combining workmen's boots, beards and moustaches with very feminine dresses and full make-up.

In Europe the drag queens' performances slowly spread in the postwar period, influenced by news of those in the United States. They first took hold in Northern Europe and then arrived in Italy around 1950 (Marcasciano 2002: 23 ff.).[12] In the beginning they functioned as an exotic performance in night clubs for straight audiences, for example the famous Coccinelle in France, or the presence of spectacular transvestites in films such as *La Dolce Vita* by Federico Fellini. Then, in the late 1960s, they started to represent a subcultural institution linked with the wider youth, minority rights and countercultural movements of the period. In the USA, the spirit of the 1930 Drag Ball was revived in the late 1980s, when groups of gay men and transvestites bonded in 'houses' with an older drag queen as their 'mother' or leader (Cole 2000: 52–53). These houses vied with each other in 'walks' at house balls. In some sections the contestants competed in gender 'realism' categories. In others the aim was the usual camp inversion of gender identities. The most famous event of the house balls was the so called *voguing*: a supermodel walk, in which each drag queen had to sashay down the runway imitating his favourite superstar model while wearing an *haute couture* gown.[13]

Into the Field

The history of the figure of the drag queen helps us to understand that the acts and practices of my interlocutors are not the products of single individual who possesses a rare and deviant 'gift'. They are, rather, the joint product of all the people who cooperate via the canons, standards and conventions of the drag queen's art world to bring their performance into existence.

That's also true for their visual skills. Although it is rooted in a common human biological substrate, the ability to pick up certain kinds of visual information is not innate nor arbitrary. Optical clues are selected and become evidence only after they have undergone an elaborate social process of transformation. In this way, what a drag queen thematises and focalises in his environment depends on 'what makes sense' in terms of his art world.

I first realised the existence of this social division of visual and cognitive work during my initial period of acquaintance with the drag queen's world.

Not being a homosexual, and without any training in the gay and drag queen world, I wasn't able at the beginning to posit myself in the 'point of view' of Carlo and his colleagues. A good example can be found in my inability to tune my 'hetero' or 'straight' visual skills with their notion of *bellezza* (beauty).[14] Not only did I lose the citation-effect of numerous performances but, in a more radical way, my eyes failed to focus on the same things selected by the eyes of the drag queens. For me the beauty canon was linked with the approximation in form and movement to standard contemporary mass media images of seductive and attractive women: thin, young, with adolescent hips, small or medium-sized breasts, light make-up, little jewellery, and so on. But for drag queens their sense of beauty was not a real-life social category but a theatrical one and it was linked to the old visual standard of the USA in the period from 1940 to 1970, the years in which the drag queen institution blossomed. In this way, a drag queen is a 'beauty' when exhibiting a slender body with the appearance of large breasts and wide hips, a face with 'good' bone structure, skin that seems soft but is heavily and dramatically made-up, jewellery (especially earrings), a long-haired wig, a gown (preferably low-cut and floor length), and, invariably, high-heeled shoes.

A second, and less obvious, case of sociocultural 'blindness' comes from the reaction of Arturo, an upper-middle-class gay who guided me in some of my tours of the homosexual world of Verona. Obviously, an art world does not have clear boundaries but is organised along a sort of continuum. If we consider all the people who are linked with an art world we see that they range from people totally involved to those that are only marginally related to it. As I've just said, not all the self-defined gays of Verona appreciate the camp logic of the drag queen art world. A lot of them are consequently unfamiliar with its style, models and canons. For this reason, it was not strange that, after our first drag queen show, Arturo told me he was a little ashamed of the lack of taste of the show and preoccupied about the bad reputation it might throw on the other more 'straight' gay men of the city. What is more interesting is that he was initially unable – like me – to interpret the visual clues in the appropriate way. At the beginning, we picked up the optical array offered by the drag queens as visible signs of a hidden reality, something that refers to an inner state of femininity of deep private nature. But, for Arturo, as for the greater part of contemporary Euro-American homosexuals, to be gay is not to be a 'female soul trapped in a man's body' but rather to have a desire for persons of the same sex (for a wide historical and cultural comparative perspective see Murray 2000). Thus, to see a gay show apparently infused by this old stereotype was for him a source of rage and contempt. It was only after seeing various other shows and talking with Madame Sisi and his colleagues that our visual landscape began to be linked in the right way with the social practice and cultural experience of the drag queen's art world. In this way, the first thing we learned was that for a drag queen the visual landscape is plain, simple and one-dimensional: it is something that refers only to the ability he possesses as a skilled performer and not to his private condition. The second thing we learned – deeply linked to the first one – was the ironic and subversive role attributed by this female impersonation. The use of the old stereotype was not a mirror or an endorsement of its content but an ironic subversion of the whole system of gender roles that sustain it (especially in the past).

In other words, wherever a visual skill exists, it defines various kinds of boundaries: on the one hand, those of acceptable art, on the other hand, the one of sociocultural belonging.

Camp as a Way of Seeing

As indicated by the examples above, to judge, appreciate and perform a certain drag show it is necessary not only to learn various kinds of performing abilities (singing, dancing, story-telling, and so on) but also to develop what Charles Goodwin has called a 'professional vision': a certain kind of visual ability capable of selecting the relevant feature of a particular professional domain and understanding their specific meaning (Goodwin 1994).[15]

This is especially true for an outsider art like that of my interlocutors. Given the long history of stigmatisation that characterises homosexual acts and persons in Europe and the United States, gays, lesbians and transgenders have developed a strong need for secrecy, hidden codes and protective behaviours to exclude 'straights' (for example Humphrey 1970).[16]

Following this lead, in the course of the fieldwork I noticed that the visual skills of my troupe of drag queens involved an informal and continuous training centred on their visual landscape, the optical array offered by the ordinary environment.[17] Specifically, it was possible to identify three main areas linked with their visual education. These are, in the order in which I shall present them: everyday world, media and artefacts, acts and performance.

The Everyday World

The first models for the performance of Madame Sisi and his colleagues are the women they encounter in the course of their *everyday life*. Obviously, the feminine style used by the drag queen doesn't reflect the actual look of any specific woman but emphasises in a camp way 'pieces' derived from various kinds of feminine *habitus* (rural, urban, wealthy, popular). In general, the main features are the repertory of words and expressions ('cute', 'divine', rising intonation), the stock of gestures and postures (indirect glance, face inclination, hands fluttering) and the ways of dressing (vamp, teenager, housewife). More specifically, what is important is that the everyday and distributed nature of these informal models often opens the way for a strong regional and biographical inflection in the performances. For example, one of the female characters impersonated by Roberto, from Bologna (in the Emilia-Romagna region), is *Virginia* (often used as a pun on virginity), a women with a strong Emilian regional identity. In Italy, women from this region are represented as very hot, fiery, direct, buxom (a lot of sexually active women in the Italian cinema are modelled on this stereotype). The same can be said for *Miss Titty* (often used as a pun on *tette*, a popular Italian word for *teats*), a female character impersonated by Lorenzo, from Mogliano Veneto, a small town in the centre of the Veneto region. In this case the regional female stereotype is the *servetta* (little house servant) a thin woman of gentle and delicate physical traits with a sharp, unblushing and strategic intelligence hidden behind her shy and servient attitude.[18]

Acts and Performances

As usual in every art world, the most obvious stock of models and standards is offered by the 'works' produced inside the art world itself, in this case the act performed by members of the troupe themselves and by other drag queens (Figure 3.2).

Usually, the roles acted by drag queens centre around two main figures: the glamour drag (young, sophisticated and well mannered) and the comic drag (vulgar, ridiculous and excessive). Moreover there are four basic types of performance: dancing, singing, glamour and comedy. Although performers tend to specialise in certain recognised artistic numbers, these are overlapping categories. For example, even those who sing serious songs must always look glamorous to a certain extent, and glamour queens generally choose the 'vocalist' form to display their look and postures.

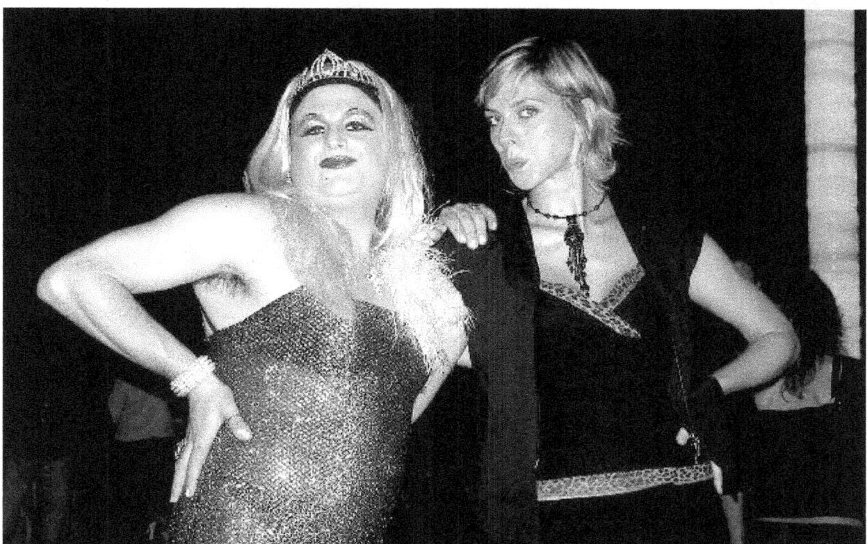

Figure 3.2 *Roberto/Virginia poses with a girl from the audience during a pause in the performance.* (Photo: F. Ronzon)

The emphasis on skill among singers gives them very high prestige.[19] The repertory of songs is usually taken from old pop and disco music. In general they are linked by factors such as reference to gay icons or canons, double-meaning lyrics, carnivalesque music. All dance acts mimic some style of female dancing but the most common is the 'strip'. The trick in stripping is to look and move as much like a 'real' woman as possible and then, as a climax, to reveal the male identity.

In the end, almost all successful performers have evolved a style based on the contrast of glamour and comedy within a single act.[20] Specifically, there are two principal kinds of comedy: slapstick and stand-up comedy. Slapstick utilises gross comic effects, usually visual. The performers attempt to make themselves look as ridiculous as possible. Stand-up comedy, on the other hand, relies mainly on verbal agility; as is frequently recognised, Euro-American homosexual subcultures give high value to incisive verbal wit (for a general overview of the topic see Leap 1995).

All the performances, my informants always contended, have a double aim: one is to make people laugh, the other is to make people think. Although it is never offered through explicit statements, the camp logic which informs the dress, objects and postures selected for the shows is directed at poking fun at the official gender *habitus*.

Media and Artefacts

At a third level, the visual skills of my troupe of drag queens were informed by various kinds of *cognitive artefacts*, media which select or emphasise on their surfaces only those features of the events relevant for their aims and interests. When these external scaffoldings are used as mediating artefacts they propagate certain specific canons, standards and protocols, routing the way of seeing of their users in a wider social matrix.

The first example is the case of the famous *gay icons*: images of celebrities of music, cinema and television used by the drag queen as examples of their camp aesthetics. In particular, Madame Sisi and his colleagues tend to mimic female performers who (a) are widely known, (b) have a highly individualistic and mannered style and (c) are well-liked by the gay community. It is important to note that if the first two criteria are very general, the last one introduces a sub-cultural filter which makes a selection based on various distinctive aspects: unnatural or androgynous look, explicit sympathy for the gay movement, explicit or implicit content of their art performance, personal sexual tendencies (real or hypothesised), and so on.

Another example can be found in the explicit visual models of international drag queens offered by gay magazines and advertisements. If you look at the most important Italian gay magazines such as *Babilonia* (glossy and expensive), *Pride* (printed on normal paper and available for free in every gay bar and disco) or *Il Cassero* (the monthly free magazine of a famous gay place and association in Bologna, also the national centre of ARCI-Gay, the most

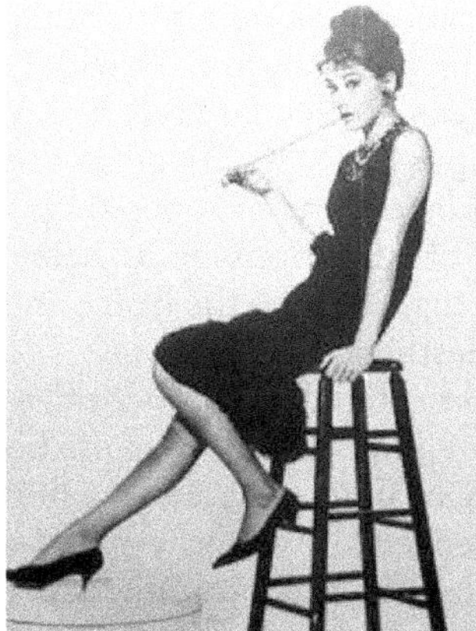

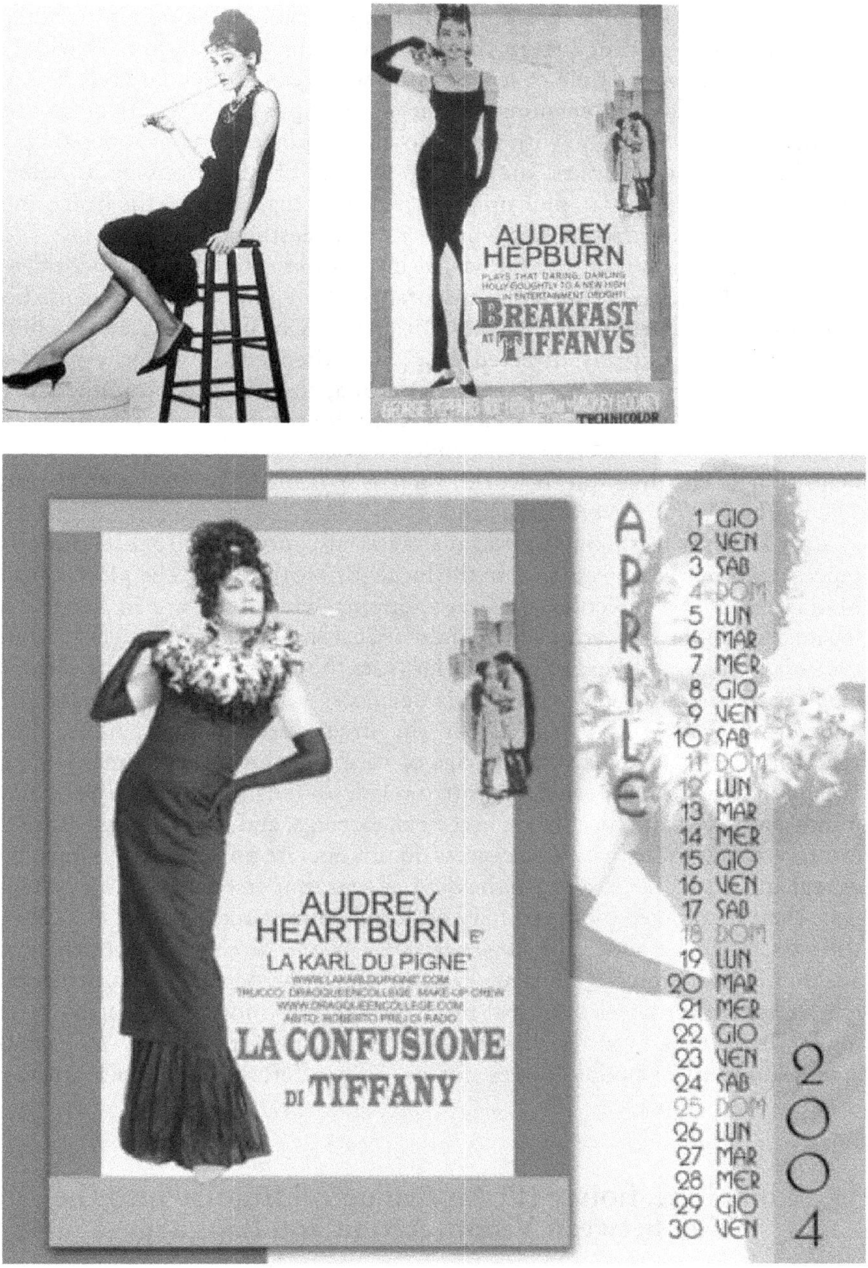

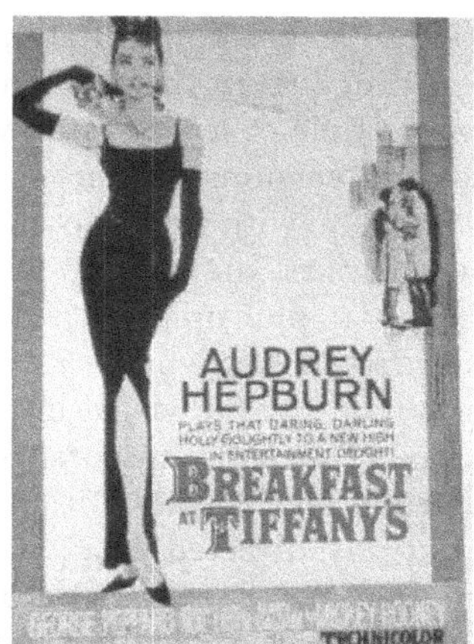

Figure 3.3 *A page from the Italian drag queen calendar, 2004.* The juxtaposition between the photo (a), the poster (b) and the drag interpretation (c) highlights the various levels of image abstraction and construction and the need for a complementary visual skill.

important gay political association in Italy), you will note a number of drag queen images that range from three to eleven in each edition. A widely circulating item at the time of my research was a camp calendar (Figure 3.3) that reproduced camp versions of famous film posters. The effect of this implicit visual comparison with well-known film posters was considered very useful by my interlocutors: the intentional play of 'variations on a theme' helped them learn how to pick up the visual clues that connote the ironic and subtle art of passing from a 'straight' to a 'camp' aesthetic.

The same can be said for the visual inspiration offered by the world of audio-visual material (TV, DVD, videotapes). One important source of this kind was represented by the recently born pay-TV channel GAY.TV, the first Italian network entirely directed at a gay audience. Moreover, even in a Catholic and provincial city such as Verona, the big French multi-store FNAC (renowned for its gay-friendly attitude) exhibits a shelf completely dedicated to gay, lesbian and transgender movies, a lot of which have as their main subject the drag queen world, such as *Priscilla. The Queen of Desert*, *The Rocky Horror Picture Show*, and so on.

Last but not least, one important material source of visual learning is represented by the objects sold in the local gay erotic-shop. The place where Madame Sisi and his colleagues go shopping when they are in Verona is located inside the hangar of a huge industrial storehouse in a hidden street in the industrial area of Verona (but not far from the centre). Among the various black erotic dresses and paraphernalia one notes at first glance the bright and colourful accessories intended for the drag queen performances. The repertory includes items such as wigs of various colours, heavy make-up, a large number of high-heeled shoes (from chic to fetish platform styles), and minor paraphernalia (necklaces, bracelets, earrings, and so on). In this case it is interesting to note that these objects do not operate only as models but also as real and actual constraints to the drag queens' impersonations. In a certain way, they are obliged by the paucity of 'look' options and resources to orient their dress choice and relative visual skills in one direction rather than in another. Thus, we can say that, even in the niche of the gay subcultural market, the macrolevel of global mass production (most of the items were made in China for multinational companies) produces a partial standardisation of people's lives not only by offering models but also by limiting their choices.

'Look here, honey !!': An Ecological Inquiry into the Link between Vision, Action and Language

In the above section I have shown how many of the items, canons and models that inform the visual skills of Madame Sisi and his colleagues are not acquired through official and formal teaching sessions but are found 'out there' in the world, in the visual clues detectable in their ordinary environment. But to pick up this informal environmental information, my interlocutors behave not in a private manner but in a highly social one. This is particularly obvious if we remember the long historical tradition of balls, parades and beauty contests operating in the art world of the drag queen from its inception. During my fieldwork I frequently heard the most expert part of the public judging or talking about the performances of Madame Sisi and his colleagues. In the same way, I often caught members of the troupe hotly debating such topics as beauty, appropriate dress and make-up, good performances and audience reaction.

In all these situations the visual landscape was included in the actions of my subjects as part of an informal *modelling* process: an interaction that put into focus a slice of the world as a resource useful for giving the female impersonator something to 'do' or a form to work within or against. When two or more drag queens gather around a visual landscape worthy of attention for their aim and interest they face the task of identifying its relevant features, their meaning and role in everyday situations. In the course of this interactive organisation of vision, various kinds of discursive practice are used by Madame Sisi and his colleagues to shape, judge and organise the stimuli in the domain subject to their professional scrutiny.

Obviously, with different visual landscapes, different optical features become relevant, yet it was possible to note the presence of some patterns of interaction. At the wider level the interaction was structured by a social logic based on overlapping criteria of age and rank: questions are always posed to the most expert members of the troupe by the younger one as he seeks to learn more about it.[21] While the above social logic can be found in all appropriate encounters, it don't exhaust the 'whole' analysis.

At a more specific level of analysis, it can be said that the verbal interaction between Madame Sisi and his colleagues sustained two kinds of social regulation of vision: (1) *coding*, which transforms phenomena observed in a specific setting into the objects of knowledge that animate the discourse of the drag queen's art world; (2) *highlighting*, which makes the specific phenomena occurring in the complex perceptual field of Madame Sisi and his colleagues salient by marking them in some fashion (see also Goodwin 1994).

At a final and even more particularised level of inquiry, it must be said that the real structure of drag queen interactive talk also includes talk patterns in which different conversational devices propel the exchange for variable periods of time. In this perspective, as well recognised by Knorr-Cetina in her ethnographic analysis of shop talk in science laboratories, three patterns of talk are particularly notable for their role as general inference-producing devices. They are, in the order in which I present them: procedural implicature, optical induction and oppositional device (Knorr-Cetina and Amann 1988: 97).

Procedural Implicature

Procedural implicature is an interrogation carried out by drag queens to produce features of the history of the visual phenomenon which aid in its interpretation and in framing its relevant feature. The exchange consists of a series of question-–answer and/or assertion–confirmation adjacency pairs of utterances in which the first utterance constrains the second (as in a question which demands an answer), which accesses and makes public indexical information from eyewitnesses of a phenomenon. In these situations the expert is consulted in an interactive, stepwise fashion as a living archive of the details which constitute the landscape of vision. The pattern may be followed by a conclusion in the form of an interpretation (this means...) or a performance recommendation (I would..., you've got to...). The following example is part of a longer interrogatory series which attempts to establish if the new look of Carlo is *divino* (divine; in the emphatic effeminate jargon of drag queens it implies a sort of theatrical glamour) or more ordinary. The procedural inquiry is initiated after Carlo indicates the part of dress that best connotes this value:

Carlo: Do you like my new look ? This turban makes me feel very *divina*.

Andrea: Yes, it's beautiful ! How did it come about?

Carlo: I don't know. It reminds me an old woman who lived next to my parents. She was a sort of aristocrat. I always saw her walking with an aura of mystery. Very exotic ...

Andrea: Hu, hu ... But don't you think that's all too 'quiet' to be really *divino*?

Carlo: No, my dear, try to imagine: powder, eyeliner and a whispery voice. A music like 'As time goes by' [from the famous film *Casablanca*] in the background while I enter the stage. Then I start to tell stories with sophisticated aplomb ... but with a lot of double meaning. And ... , yes, and when I use double meaning I change my voice from female falsetto to a rough male slang. Obviously, I'm talking of a high-class performance, not of some kind of *Star Wars* [George Lucas's famous science fiction film]. You know ... something like Garbo or Marilyn [very famous gay icons]. And it's little things like this turban that give this look its special allure. Oh, honey ..., but you're so young [exhaling with a blasè posture].

From the transcript it is easy to notice that this device is employed to derive non-obvious conclusions from a mute visual landscape by means of an inquiry into the procedures through which these outcomes have come about. Specifically, an answer to a procedural question may take more than one turn and rely on more than one interlinked level of exegesis.

Optical Induction

Optical induction can be seen as a hybrid between visual operations and conversations. In this situation, it is the reference at the visual landscape itself which prompts clues towards the 'right' way of seeing. The operation consists in large part in visual operations carried out through talk. The linguistic means, however, are not question–answer adjacency pairs or assertions and confirmations, but sequences which include formulations of details of the visual landscape mixed with interpretations.

As Madame Sisi and his colleagues inspect visual features of their look, posture and performance, as they pay attention to and compare the details of these features, they establish and reject candidates' identification of visual clues, and they do so in the sequential fashion typical of collaborative talk. The following example centres around the visual landscape offered by a photo of various American drag queens in a gay magazine and it illustrates how drag queens' visual analysis leads to certain interpretations and how these interpretations in turn give rise to a new round of visual operations:

Luigi: Look at this one, honey [points to the photo in the magazine] what a difference! He has a lot of charm. This other here doesn't even have half a shade of the first.

Andrea: Mmm, what a snake! If you pay attention it is clear that this effect is a photographer choice. The crux is his nose, his eyes. You don't have to be absorbed by the dress only. Pay attention at his ephebic face ... What an angel !!

Luigi: No, *stellina* [little star, a sentimental nickname, here pronounced with a sharp ironical inflection]. Can't you see the lipstick? You must agree with me that this heart-shaped mouth is absolutely out of fashion ... And those pink stockings don't have anything to do with the light green of the shoes. Either you dare to be a real *mignotta* [prostitute, but usually employed for bad women] or it's better to change your character.

Andrea: I know. In fact he's not trying to imitate a vamp but a sort of yé-yé girl like Caterina Caselli.[22] Do you remember?

Which of the visual clues is the relevant one is not obvious from what one sees in the visual landscape. Drag queens must work out the visual traces and they do it by shifting their attention to various parts of the visual image, comparing the signs which appear on the surface, taking some signs at face value, and going back and forth between the clues and the wider logic of their art world. Occasionally, as happens in this example, opinions clash. On such occasions another routine of talk overlaps and takes over the conversation.

Oppositional device

The third and last interactional strategy for vision is the *oppositional device*: the turning point where the exchange become adversarial. To some extent, oppositive patterns of interaction 'feed upon' or overlay other conversational patterns (they are, in fact, not only adversarial but also argumentative). They often start by one drag queen objecting to the proposal made by another. They continue by participants arguing with and negotiating about each other's accounts of issues raised. In the following example, a quarrel between Carlo and Lorenzo on the theme of *trans* drag (from transvestite, with the meaning of 'deviance', self-expression without conformity to the drag queen art world's canon), such segments are found throughout the transcript. The visual object of contention was an unknown female impersonator in the audience of a gay disco-pub in Padova (a city near Verona with a lively gay world) where my troupe of drag queens was performing at the time:

Carlo: Hey, take a look at that drag! [pointing with the head at a man in the left corner of the room]
Lorenzo: Oh, My god, no! [with a loud effeminate tone] He has nothing to do with us!! He's a *trans*!!
Carlo: You're wrong. He's not a simple *marchetta* [whore in jargon, but with a mellow judegment].[23] You can see it from his eyes.
Lorenzo: Don't make fun of me. If he's a drag, I'm the Virgin Mary. He's so naif.
Carlo: He wears good. He's very griffed.
Lorenzo: Yes, but here we are in the rich northeast, my dear! Not in Sicily!!
Carlo: Listen! [with the index and the whole arm pointing in a theatrical way at the subject] I tell you that he's a drag. If he had been a *trans*, he would have been much rougher. Maybe, he's a 'tacky' drag [cheap, shoddy, a poor or low-class quality imitation of a high quality model or standard] but he is surely not a *trans*.
Lorenzo: Oh, shut up! Anyway I would never have him as a partner on the stage.
Carlo: Oh, yes! That's true, absolutely!!

In this case it is worth noting that the point of such adversarial dialogue is not simply the persuasion of one participant by another or the negotiation of firmly held opinions until a compromise is reached. First, Carlo and Lorenzo develop their contribution as they go along in response to problem features they become aware of. Second, their adversarial exchange does not end with an agreement but nonetheless produces a conclusion on which participants can proceed.[24]

Conclusions

Mind, as Gregory Bateson always insisted, is not 'in the head' as opposed to 'out there in the world'. It is instead immanent in the active, perceptual engagement of organism and environments (Bateson 1973). To investigate the impact of this ecological perspective on the topic of vision, I have chosen some examples from the art world of an Italian troupe of drag queens because their role as specialists (artist) and marginals (homosexuals) offers powerful insights into the ways in which visual skill is socially and personally acquired and applied in everyday situations. To conclude, I think there are at least four ecological lessons to be derived from the ethnographic case I presented above.

The first is that the ability to look at the world from a drag queen 'point of view' is not only linked to their biological perceptual system but to their ability to learn and apply a certain kind of attention.

The second is that the visual skills possessed by my troupe of drag queens are not based on some mental or language-like internal 'social representation' that bears some complex relation with the outside world but, rather, are part of a social activity that is embedded in the nexus of ongoing relations between persons and the world. In other words, these skills are inseparable from the actual biography and situated activity of their owners as part of a process wherein both persons and the settings in which they act (other persons included) continually come into being, each in relation to the other.

The third refers to the role that language exerts on vision. As they examine their visual landscape, the drag queens begin a series of verbal exchanges. Thus, the resulting perceptual identification is not just the product of language, it is the product of conversational talk (Goodwin 1993; Lynch 1985). When embodied in talk, seeing is interactively accomplished: the process does not involve a hypothetical translation into a generalised system of signs, nor an interpretative process of individual conceptual decoding. Instead, the process has an interactive structure and this implies that visual analysing talk is attached to the objects which are the subject of the exchanges. Drag queens interact not only with each other but also with the object to which they attach their comments. They tend to return repeatedly to the same visual landscape to discuss the contents of their speeches, an act made possible by the continued mutual accessibility of participants while they observe their optical referent. It is the world which integrates the series of exchanges, not the continuity of the speakers. Participants do not seem to resolve issues raised by the features of their environments once and for all. Instead, they repeatedly 'visit' the problems, thus continually reopening the cases.

The fourth and last lesson concerns what we can call the social life of visual skill. If we compare a drag queen's visual skill with that of an outsider, their peculiarities show us how things which seem ordinary in the making of professional drag queen vision need not to be that way at all; how things could be looked at differently; and what the result of doing it differently would be. When these skills are used the social effects of this distinction become clear. On the one hand, visual skills function to establish expertise, social identity and solidarity with group members. On the other hand, exclusive visual skills function as an invisible boundary to newcomers and non-members of the group. Even more interesting, however, is the fact that this cleavage can be highly ambiguous and context dependent. In fact, the visual skills of Madame Sisi and his colleagues provide a means of simultaneously employing and subverting the dominant standard of gender. In this way, the visual skills linked with the explicit and conscious artistic production of camp stereotyped effeminacy diffuse the derogatory power of heterosexist assumptions about queer behaviour. The camp logic used by drag queens in their appropriation of symbols of hegemonic gender standard leaves space for an ironic reworking of their meaning. As Judith Butler epitomises with great subtlety, the parody or imitative effect of the drag queens works neither to copy nor to emulate heterosexuality, but rather to expose heterosexuality as an incessant and panicked imitation of its own naturalised idealisation and essentialisation (Butler 1991). This suggests that the presence of a dominant hegemonic variety may not always represent complicity or collaboration with the dominant social group. The use and appropriation of aspects of the dominant subcultural variety may actually serve as a means of inversion and contestation of the domination symbolised by the variety.

In synthesis, these four reflections seem to suggest that in order to put the topic of vision under ecological analysis we are required to rethink the whole enterprise of cognitive ethnography from what Jean Lave has called an 'outdoor psychology': a theory of mind that would take as its unit of analysis 'the whole person in action, acting within the settings of that activity' (Lave 1988:17). Contrary to the axioms of 'classic' cognitive anthropology, the intersubjectivity and communion of experience that lies at the heart of drag queens' socialised visual skills does not depend upon the organisation of sensory data, initially private to each perceiver, in terms of an ideal system of collective and language-like internal representation. Rather, their sociality is given from the start in the direct perceptual involvement of fellow participants in a shared environment. As suggested by Tim Ingold, using one's body in the same way as others in the same environment is what makes possible ordinary social life – and anthropological fieldwork – for it allows different individuals as well as individuals coming from different places to inhabit a basic level of experience (Ingold 2000: 167).

What the visual skills of Madame Sisi and his colleagues say to cognitive ethnography is that to investigate the interactive organisation of cognition we need to focus on a wider reality than the one offered by the isolated mind or language; and that this world is not naked but 'dragged' with bodies, artefacts, practical expertise and social institutions.

Notes

1 The research was funded by CRRPS/Veneto Region as part of a media project of sensibilisation of young gays to HIV risks. I would like to thank all those whose help made my research possible. In particular, I would like to thank G. Zardini of *Circolo Pink*, Z. Menegazzi of *Urano-Arci Gay* for their help as insiders and gatekeepers in the course of the fieldwork.

2 This move represents a departure from the main tradition of cognitive anthropology. This subfield emerged in the 1950s as an alternative to neo-Freudism and behaviourism implicit in the works of the 'culture and personality' school, alongside the development of the digital computer. Its founding axioms are that people come to know what is 'out there' in the world by representing it in the mind, in the form of abstract 'mental models', and that such representations are the result of various kinds of computational processes working upon information received by the senses. The functioning of the mind, then, can be loosely

compared to the operation of a computer program; and the relation between mind and brain to that between software and the hardware in which it is installed (for a general introduction see de Andrade 1995).

3 For an exemplary critical comparison between ecological and representational cognitive theory see the hard debate between Fodor and Pylyshyn (1981) and Reed et al. (1981) on the pages of Cognition.

4 It is important to highlight the difference between a *queen* and a *drag queen* (Newton 1972). 'Queen' is a label that refers to the ordinary, non-professional male transvestite. 'Drag queen' refers instead to the expert professional female impersonator. In the last twenty years there has been a huge increment of ethnographic and anthropological research on the themes of transvestitism and transgenderism. Some are organised in a comparative style (for example: Herdt 1996; Petra Ramet 1996). Others consist of book-length fieldwork monographs (for example: Bolin 1988; Kulick 1998; Nanda 1999; Prieur 1998; Young 2000).

5 According to Erving Goffman, the term 'stigma' refers to an attribute that is deeply discrediting (1963:3). Attributes that can cause an individual or groups of individuals to be discredited are physical and/or mental handicaps, terminal illness, class background, education, race or ethnicity, as well as sexual and gender orientation.

6 It is important to remember that an art world consists of the cooperative activities of its members, not as a structure or formal organisation.

7 It is a pun on the sophistication of French names and language (Sissi) and the usual 'si, si' (in English: yes, yes) with which Carlo punctuates his sentences.

8 Carlo has been running nightclubs and discothèques for sixteen years. He has run the Art since 1987. As Madame Sisi, he also conducts a talk show from 1 p.m. to 2 p.m. for a local radio station of mid-range.

9 In Verona there are two specifically gay discos: the disco-pub Romeo's and the big open discothèque Limelight.

10 In more formal language, we could say that the logic of 'camp' implies the creation of an ambiguous relationship between the referential meaning of an appearance and the intended or inferred meaning. Some researchers compare this attitude with the practice of signifying an ironical rhetorical device in African-American English (see in Leap 1995).

11 Not all gay men have a favourable view of the drag balls. In many cases their views are similar to those of the men who objected to overtly effeminate gay men. Anything of a semi-legal nature which aids in breaking down the veils of secrecy and in bringing the homosexual life into the open is desirable. This criticism is coupled with the belief that the drag queen panders to an old naïve stereotype of homosexuality: that a man who desires another man is a sort of female in disguise.

12 It should be noted that the Italian drag queen tradition is a completely 'foreign' cultural import. There are no links with the older local tradition of 'femminielli' in Naples (South Italy).

13 In the USA this was, in some respects, a reaction to the ultra macho image of gay men diffused in the late 1970s and early 1980s by the clone and leather gay style. For an updating of the Italian gay macho situation see Ronzon (2004).

14 For a wider series of reflections on the various kinds of social links existing between beauty on one side and gender-power on the other, see Ballerino Cohen et al. (1996).

15 Other senses like touch or smell are not relevant or thematised. The spatial distance between the stage and the audience is the main reason for the visual bias of this art world.

16 Steven Epstein (1990) makes an analogy between gay and lesbian identity and ethnic identity. In Epstein's analogy of ethnicity as a corollary to gay and lesbian identities he states that 'gay communities have developed a variety of cultural forms which, despite the considerable internal variation, serve to unify those communities' (1990: 280).

17 For a wider reflection on the ecological and relational quality of the landscape see Hirsch and O'Hanlon (1995).

18 From a wider point of view, it is possible to find traces of this regional model of femininity even in the art world of the 'Commedia dell'Arte' of Luca Goldoni.

19 Of course, there is a basic distinction between the true vocalist and the recorded vocalist in that the latter only mimic the act of singing (using playback) as a basic format for their performance.

20 This is especially true for older drag queens: in order to continue they must temper the glamour impersonation with more and more humour. Carlo is a good example of this category.

21 In contrast to the findings of many students of institutional encounters such as medical interviews, calls to the police or classroom interaction (for example West 1983), the 'drag' inquirers do not appear to dominate the encounter by placing limits on the placements and content of recipients' responses. On the contrary, it was usually the person questioned who controlled as a valuable good the relevant information, whereas the questioner sought to obtain a share in this good.

22 A famous beat Italian singer. In the 1960s she was the interpreter of Nessuno mi può giudicare (Nobody can judge me), a song now taken as a sort of battle hymn by the Italian gay movement and frequently used also by drag queens for their more assertive performances. In the gossip of the Italian gay community, this singer is also reputed a 'hidden' lesbian.

23 The link between a *trans* and a *marchetta* operated by my interlocutors is based on their shared assumption that the *trans* earn their living mainly from prostitution and not from artistic performance, as the drag queen does.

24 It is interesting to note that this situation is in contrast to the preference for agreement that researchers encounter in other institutional situations, for example in doctor–patient interaction (Brown and Levinson 1978; Sachs 1973).

References

Ballerino Cohen, C., R. Wilk and B. Stoeltje, eds. 1996. *Beauty Queens on the Global Stage: Gender, Contests, and Power*. New York and London: Routledge.

Bateson, G. 1973. *Steps to an Ecology of Mind*. London: Fontana.

Becker, H.S. 1982. *Art Worlds*. Berkeley: University of California Press.

Bolin, A. 1988. *In Search of Eve: Transexual Rites of Passage*. Westport: Bergin & Garvey.

Brown, P. and Levinson, S. 1978. 'Universal in Language Usage: Politeness Phenomena', in *Questions and Politeness*, ed. E. Goody. Cambridge: Cambridge University Press.

Butler, J. 1991. 'Imitation and Gender Subordination', in *Inside/Out Lesbian Theories, Gay Theories*, ed. D. Fuss. London: Routledge.

Chauncey, G. 1994. *Gay New York: Gender, Urban Culture, and the Making of Gay Male World, 1890–1940*. New York: Basic Books.

Cole, S. 2000. *'Don We now Our Gay Apparel'. Gay Men's Dress in the Twentieth Century.* Oxford and New York: Berg.

De Andrade, R. 1995. *The Development of Cognitive Anthropology*. Cambridge: Cambridge University Press.

Epstein, S. 1990. 'Gay Politics, Ethnic Identity: The Limits of Social Constructivism', in *Form of Desire: Sexual Orientation and Social Constructionist Controversy*, ed. E.W. Stein. New York: Garland Publishing, Inc.

Fodor, J.A. and Z.W. Pylyshyn, 1981. 'How Direct is Visual Perception?: Some Reflections on Gibson's Ecological Approach', *Cognition* 9: 139–96.

Gibson, J.J. 1979. *The Ecological Approach to Visual Perception*. Boston: Houghton Mifflin.

Goffman, E. 1963. *Stigma: Notes on the Management of Spoiled Identity*. Englewood Cliffs: Prentice-Hall.

Goodwin, C. 1993 'The Blackness of Black: Color Categories as Situated Practice', in *Discourse, Tools and Reasoning: Essays on Situated Cognition*, eds. L.B. Resnick, R. Saljo, C. Pontecorvo and B. Burge. Berlin and New York: Springer, 111–140.

—— 1994. 'Professional Vision', *American Anthropologist* 3: 606–33

—— 1996. 'Transparent Vision', in *Interaction and Grammar*, eds. E. Ochs, E.A. Schegloff, S. Thompson. Cambridge: Cambridge University Press.

Grasseni, C. and F. Ronzon, 2004. *Pratiche e Cognizione. Note di Ecologia della Cultura*. Roma: Meltemi.

Herdt, G. ed. 1996. *Third Sex, Third Gender. Beyond Sexual Dimorphism in Culture and History*. New York: Zone Books.

Hirsch, E. and M. O'Hanlon, eds. 1995 *The Anthropology of Landscape. Perspectives on Place and Space*. Clarendon Press: Oxford.

Humphrey, L. 1970. *Tearoom Trade. Impersonal Sex in Public Places*. New York: Aldine de Gruyter.

Ingold, T. 2000. *The Perception of the Environment. Essays in Livelihood, Dwelling and Skill*, London and New York: Routledge.

Knorr-Cetina, K. and K. Amann, 1988. 'The Fixation of (visual) Evidence', in *Representation in Scientific Practice*, eds. M. Lynch and S. Woolgar. Cambridge, Mass.: MIT Press.

Kulick, D. 1998. *Travestì. Sex, Gender and Culture among Brazilian Transgendered Prostitutes*. Chicago and London: University of Chicago Press.

Lave, J. 1988. *Cognition in Practice*. Cambridge: Cambridge University Press.

Leap, W.L., ed. 1995. *Beyond the Lavender Lexicon: Authenticity, Imagination and Appropriation in Lesbian and Gay Languages*. Newark: Gordon and Breach Publishers.

Lynch, M. 1985. *Art and Artefact in Laboratory Science: A Study of Shop Work and Shop Talk in a Research Laboratory*. London: Routledge & Kegan Paul.

Marcasciano, P., ed. 2002. *Tra le Rose e le Viole. La Storia e le Storie di Transessuali e Travestiti*. Roma: ManifestoLibri.

Murray, S.O. 2000. *Homosexualities*. Chicago: University of Chicago Press.

Nanda, S. 1999. *The Hijras of India. Neither Man nor Woman*. Belmont: Wadsworth.

Newton, E. 1972. *Mother Camp: Female Impersonators in America*. Chicago and London: University of Chicago Press.

Petra Ramet, S., (ed.) 1996. *Gender Reversals & Gender Cultures. Anthropological and Historical Perspectives*. London and New York: Routledge.

Prieur, A. 1998. *Mema's House. On Transvestites, Queens, and Machos*. Chicago and London: University of Chicago.

Reed, E.S. 1988. *James J. Gibson and the Psychology of Perception*. New Haven: Yale University Press

Reed, E.S., M.T. Turvey, R.E. Shaw and W.M. Mace, 1981. 'Ecological Laws of Perceiving and Acting: In Reply to Fodor and Phylyhin', *Cognition* 9: 237–304.

Ronzon, F. 2004. 'Pelle & Metallo. Identità di Genere, Omosessualità e Cultura Materiale nel Moto Leather Club Veneto (Italia)', *DiPav Quaderni, Semestrale di psicologia e antropologia culturale* 9: 63–80.

Sachs, H. 1973. 'Current Research in Conversational Analysis: The Performance for Agreement'. Paper presented at the Summer Institute for Linguistics, Ann Arbor, Michigan.

Toren, C. 1993. 'Making History: The Significance of Childhood for a Comparative Anthropology of Mind', *Man* 2: 461–78.

West, C. 1983. 'Ask me no question ... An analysis of Queries and Replies in Physician–Patient Dialogue', in The Social *Organization of Doctoral–Patient Communication*, eds. S. Fischer and A. Todd. Washington: Center for Applied Linguistics.

Whitehouse, H. 1996. 'Jungle and Computers. Neuronal Group Selection and the Epidemiology of Representations', *Journal of the Royal Anthropological Institute* 2: 99–116.

Young, A. 2000. *Women Who Become Men. Albanian Sworn Virgins*. Oxford and New York: Berg.

Part II

Positioning Gestures of Design in Art, Architecture and Laboratories

Chapter 4

Seeing and Drawing: the Role of Play in Medical Imaging

Simon Cohn

The well-worn phrase that to 'see something is to know it' has become a customary rejoinder, confirming the degree to which sight is not only valued as the primary sense, but is so elevated that it is taken to be synonymous with thought and intellect (Bal 2003). Such a deep-rooted assumption, accompanied by its countless metaphors, is being radically critiqued by literature that claims to be turning away from the armatures of modernity. For example, some of the anthropological writings that promote the value of other sensory experiences for ethnographic interpretation and representation also refute the very idea that reality can be singularly known (Classen 1997). Certainly I am in agreement with the general claim that Western culture has been dominated by the ocularcentric paradigm (Jenks 1995), and that science in particular has been dominated by specific visual practices that both confirm as well as describe the claims made about the world, and in so doing have perpetuated the tie between image and fact (Lynch and Woolgar 1990).

However, this current volume importantly invites the inverse dictum; that frequently it is to know something that means it can ever be seen. Yet, since the very idea of knowledge is usually assumed to be solely concerned with rational thought, conscious awareness, and with knowing that one knows something, this alternative perspective appears, at least initially, to be paradoxical. The problem is that to know something so often is equated with the recognition of something that first presents itself as unknown, and it is this assumption of the temporal order that lies at the heart of the way natural sciences have tended to tell their story (Hacking 1999). In light of this apparent contradiction, I want to explore, in the context of medicine, the intertwined relationship between 'knowing' something and 'seeing it'; the ways in which what is seen comes to the fore not only because doctors and other medical experts have accumulated expectations and principles of discernment that allow a particular part of the body to come into view, but also crucially because they have acquired processes and procedures that do not, in fact, follow this linear narrative of the acquisition of knowledge. In so doing, I want to tease out some of the elements of reasoning and identification that are necessary to invest visual representations with the kind of authority that they are given, but illustrate how these come about through cultural and often mundane methods in which both knowing and seeing are experienced as aspects of the same activity.

Another key theme of this volume is the suggestion that such discrimination is not apparent to the uninitiated apprentice, but appears to be a skill acquired over time. If we cling on to a linear sense of what it might mean to come to know something, then this only adds to the intrigue, since how is it that something that apparently escapes rational identification might be imparted to the uneducated? One danger in addressing this, however, is that it can invite a romantic notion of skill as simply being some indefinite, intuitive acquisition gained in some inexplicable way from embodied, repeated action or 'raw talent', in opposition to intentional, directed judicious learning. Such a standpoint, though attractive, has itself a long cultural tradition, certainly since Rousseau, in arguments presented to defend the value of arts over the sciences, or counter the value of thought over action, and suggest that experiential learning is in some way more authentic or valid (Rousseau 1969). To avoid this, I want to argue that Western medicine, at least, has always managed to enclose this potential opposition in its very self-conscious awareness that it is both an art and a science; that it is based both on principles of subjective interpretation and on established canonical claims about the body (Bynum and Porter 1993). However, this endorsement of the 'art' of medicine is not merely a confirmation of its interpretative basis, but frequently is mobilised in the hierarchical culture of the profession and the reification of enskilment as the ultimate basis of expertise. In other words, the very intangible nature of medical proficiency, as it is constructed, and the deletion of explicit acknowledgements of ambiguity, serve to endorse the status of senior medical professionals without it ever having to be explicitly defined.

Beyond this, what is perhaps striking in modern medicine is the way in which so many innovations and new areas of expertise appear to be threatening the traditional basis of practice, setting aside the individual's skill and expertise with technologies and procedures that automate such things as visualising the body and disease (see Saunders, this volume, for such sentiment). Medical imaging has a long history, of course, but in the contemporary context the range of techniques and the ready assumptions made about their unquestionable objectivity appears to have grown exponentially (Kevles 1997). The rise of many new forms of medical imaging technologies, which are almost all based on digitalised data, might at first suggest that those facets understood to be based on intuition and indefinable processes of recognition and expectation, might be being replaced by apparatus that provides definitive and unequivocal representations. Kember (1998) suggests that in contrast with the more traditional opticism of science, digitialism is explicitly about simulation and this may well be forcing a re-evaluation of the foundations of knowledge; in other words, that in digital form, objectivity is not derived from the fixed nature of the scientific inscription, and hence might mark a 'dethroning' of Cartesian perspectivalism (Jay 1992). In so doing, the use of any notion of artistry or skill as the basis for status and seniority might itself be being eroded. However, I want to explore this a little further, and suggest that though these new systems are in many ways revolutionary, their use nevertheless has sufficient degrees of freedom to allow for a variation of this skilled vision, and hence reproduction of status, to take place. Thus, the idea of skill, though necessarily transformed to encompass new techniques of seeing and reasoning, nevertheless allows for the traditional values underpinning medical expertise to co-exist with the most advanced and apparently automated systems of visual representation.

I will first introduce some general remarks made by some surgeons from a London teaching hospital, who, as a somewhat estranged subset of medical culture, best exemplify the old 'hands-on' doctor, and who explicitly state how they draw on their own reading of the body to avoid severing a minute nerve or to identify a tumour that to the untrained eye cannot be recognised at all. Surgeons are notoriously aloof, and, according to other people that I spoke to in the hospital, exemplify an old kind of paternalistic arrogance. I want to present them briefly because they themselves actively endorse not only the idea of 'skill', but also that this is an intangible quality that only comes with experience and maturity, and that many are now lamenting the intervention of technologies between their hand and their eye. I will then contrast this with one of the burgeoning medical practices that are now free from the mess and corporeality of surgical intervention, in which the observer sits in front of a monitor while the patient is very distant and there are a multitude of technologies, procedures and other individuals in between them. Drawing on observations at an imaging site that specialises in some of the most advanced techniques to capture parts of the body in extraordinary detail, I will present the activities of these medical researchers as illustrative of an apparent contrasting context, in which the hierarchical endorsement of the acquisition of skills to interpret and make sense of what is seen is theoretically being eradicated. The point is that these techniques, by apparently being both so complicated and so automated, present the space for individuals to claim their own artistry. Ostensibly, therefore, the changing nature of a skill in vision is being replaced by a very rationalised sense of expertise based on very explicit competences that accompany the requirements of the specific technologies.

The Surgeon's Eye

Benjamin, in his most famous of essays, argues at one point that a surgeon can be contrasted with a magician or shaman, in the same way as a cameraman can be contrasted with a painter. The analogy is based on the deletion of distance: 'The magician heals a sick person by the laying on of hands; the surgeon cuts into the patient's body' in the same way as a cameraman, in contrast to a painter, penetrates rather than marvels at, the world (Benjamin 1999). For him the act of surgery, and the taking a photograph, go beneath and inevitably fragment the genuine relationship of one person with other. Yet here Benjamin is perhaps deliberately dismissing how the cautious movements of the scalpel serve to delineate the surgeon's expectations of organs and tissues as well as reveal them to her, and that the apparent collapsing of distance, can itself also be a communicative act. In conversation about this idea of distance, and the penetration of the body in surgery, one particular surgeon, sitting facing me as though I might myself perhaps be a potential patient of his one day, likened the scalpel to a pencil, declaring, 'For me, it's not about cutting or removing – though of course that's what I do. The scalpel is really about revealing something – a part of the body, an area of tissue, that I know exists beneath what I can see. I feel my way, as much as see my way. The point is that you just can't risk doing anything unless you're absolutely sure that you know what you're doing.' His self-assured comments are immediately suggestive of the entangled relationship between seeing and knowing; not only did he appear to find some sort of affirmation in the idea that what he does is an art, but his reflections avoided any emphasis that vision serves to divide and partition or that knowing is experienced simply as holding some predetermined representation of the thing (see Ingold 2000).

In discussions with other surgeons it seems that this motif is central to the way that they describe their dexterity as necessarily explorative, yet also as having to be made with confidence and certainty. In the context of this, seeing is not a single moment of apprehension, but involves an on-going combination of recognising, acknowledging and acting upon. The original surgeon went on to talk about how he drew on other senses, in particular touch – usually indirect through the equipment he used, but sometimes the more direct touch of his gloved hand, as another way of seeing: 'For me, it's all about gaining a sense of the patterns of things – every body is different, every organ is unique, and we have to navigate our way through all these variations.' Touch is presented as qualitatively different from vision precisely because it is demonstrable of proximity and the intimacy of knowing the interior of a body. Through this language experience is presented as unified, drawn from embodied sensations as well as technical knowledge. But it also served to unnerve me somewhat, the erudite descriptions somehow ensuring that I, myself, would appreciate the magic that they were able to perform.

There is another aspect to the way surgery is sometimes described. In discussions with others, a parallel emphasis is given to the body that is being operated on; as one put it, 'You have to look out for things, of course – each case is different, every organ a different shape, every blood vessel and every nerve in a different place. But you get a sense of how things are likely to be not just by concentrating on the specific, but also trying to get an overall picture.' He saw his skill not merely as one that necessarily drew from all his senses, but that also included having a sense of how the body was displaying itself. I asked him if what he was describing was the fact that he had to have a prior sense of what he would uncover, a 'mental map' of the interior of the body, before actually conducting each action: 'Yes, I suppose so. But more than that, for me surgery is a very precise art of letting the body communicate.' As we talked, his descriptions, from the acts of marking a body up, to the actual cutting, the clamping of things apart, the shifting of organs to one side, and then display of the interior, continually suggested that he understood his proficiency as intuitively enabling the body to reveal itself to him, as much as the direct result of his own invasive incisions. He said in conclusion, 'Look, I know it's a bit fanciful. And I know it's probably not really what is happening. But for me, concentrating on what I see is like listening to a patient, it's about responding to how the body shows itself to me.' Here, then, not only is skill rarefied as being the accumulation of multiple factors, but it also draws on the impression that the body itself has an agency, and under the right hands, allows itself to be seen. Yet, again, what is also striking in this portrayal is the extent to which the surgeon's abilities are presented as inescapably enigmatic and mysterious.

These sentiments, from senior surgeons, must themselves be contextualised by the rapid advance of medical technology, in which increasingly this 'art' of medicine, as it is imagined, is apparently being threatened even in the hospital theatre. There are increasing amounts of equipment that aid surgery, which is in truth usually an intervention by a team of people, rather than a single expert, as the accounts so far suggest. Much of this technology is designed to aid the team to see more. As well as endoscopies and fibre-optic torches, previously captured digital scans, replacing the role of investigative X-rays, further assist the navigation of surgery. These now allow for virtual, three-dimensional models on monitors to be continuously re-orientated and explored alongside the exploration of the body itself. In doing so, they provide a common, fixed representation of the body being operated on to be shared by the nurse, anaesthetist and often by more than one surgeon. As one surgeon mournfully put it, the very fact that just so many different people might all be scrutinising the same images meant that he felt, with so many people now involved, he sometimes 'could no longer really see what was actually going on'.

And there is yet a further development that potentially erodes the heroic depiction that some senior surgeons are keen to affirm: the increasing use of what is termed 'keyhole' surgery for many different operations – what is usually called laparoscopy for invasion into the abdomen and arthroscopic surgery when applied to the repair of joints. It's a potentially rich term, since initially it might imply an eye squinting up to a small opening, but of course, the keyhole is actually the incision through which indirect manipulations can be made, increasingly by 'remote control' electro-mechanical means. Usually a second cut allows for the introduction of an endoscope or tiny fibre-optic camera, with printouts and other forms of representation continuously generated during the course of the procedure. Not only does it mean that the size of the wound is vastly reduced, and that therefore there will be little scarring, but also it is far more efficient, since patients usually stay in hospital for much less time and may not even need general anaesthetic. Laparoscopy requires precision in different ways to the past. It requires the minute movements of instruments to sever blood vessels, or manipulate the camera, and prevents a more general assessment of the body; the surgery implied in the accounts above – the scope of vision, movements of the hand, and basis of the surgeon's skill – are framed entirely by the technical procedure, and this is interpreted as something that might threaten the basis of surgical practice.

In other words, keyhole surgery not only entirely relies on technologies to direct visualisation, but in so doing, the technique partitions the more holistic practices previously presented as 'feeling' and 'seeing' into discrete sources of information. 'I think advances in surgery have an awful lot going for them, of course', said one person still in training, 'but many of us do feel that somehow surgery is becoming quite distant. It's more and more technical, and we're having to rely on more and more other people and bits of equipment. I can't help but feel that we might be losing something here – maybe even not doing as good medicine sometimes.' There is something very evocative in this apparent nostalgia invoked by someone who actually is not yet a qualified surgeon yet who appears to reject the increasing intervention of people and objects between himself and the body being operated on. The fact that this was said by a junior medic suggests that it is not necessarily his own current proficiency that he feels is being threatened, but possibly a threat to his career aspirations. He already endorses the lack of distance between the surgeon and the body, the eye and the hand, as marking out a highly individualised sense of medical skill. And hence, the new medical technologies are conceived as competing with this indefinable abstract basis for professional status, and increasingly envisaged as denying him his own success in the future.

Distant Images

I want to contrast these sentiments with those of medical imagers who use some of the most advanced MRI (magnetic resonance imaging) techniques, and who initially appear to have no invocation of intuition, since at no point do any of them ever deal with the physical body itself. They present their activities as not requiring any skill precisely because there is a total division between themselves and the body through a multitude of technical and rationalised processes. Along a corridor of an imaging lab, well away from patients, in one of the open-plan offices, a senior neuroscientist leans over the shoulder of a more junior one, who is still doing his Ph.D. They are both staring at the flat computer screen, on which is illuminated the familiar, iconic image of a scan. 'Look,' begins the professor, waving his finger towards one part of the colourful image, 'this is clearly where most activity is located … try and clean the thing up a bit, so that these', he points to other blobs and shadows on the image, 'are not so confusing.' The junior researcher is then left alone. He puts his headphones on, isolating him once again from his peers and colleagues, to go back a few steps in the procedures of generating the image, to try out possible new thresholds and parameters. It might actually take him some weeks. He'll be using complex software packages, and a range of different graphic options, to obtain what is being asked of him. Having asked him beforehand, I know he finds the whole thing frustrating, laborious, and not quite what he expected he'd be doing: 'It just seems a black art to me', he had said. 'We are all really very different from each other, but at a statistical level it's not the case … So we are building up images in which we can tell you this voxel and this coordinate has a ninety-nine per cent chance of being in the primary visual cortex, or whatever. So you see these images are, ummm, just probability maps, and that's one of the things I'm having to get to grips with.'

Final images, averaged from a number of individual scans and then transposed onto a model of a generalised image, are the result of intertwined decisions and technical requirements between the digital data and a multitude of interim representations that can be generated from them (Blume 1992). When the actual scanning is over (it can take just a few minutes or be over an hour) the analysis begins. In truth, the image appears far from routinely, despite the intricacy of the technology. A significant tension therefore exists between the extent to which the scans are generated automatically or are the result of personal choices and decisions. Because of this, the computers, central to the very nature of the endeavour, are considered as much a hindrance as essential components, somehow getting between the researcher and what they are trying to find out. As one junior imager put it, 'The image is a sort of Ying and Yang thing … People want to find and uncover the underlying denominator – the substrate – and that's a question of commonality. But all the time there's going to be a question of variability.' This can take months and is notably protracted after the instantaneous first images that appear during the procedure. Yet, it is not merely the hours spent looking at a screen or measuring data in the well-thumbed histology reference book; frustrations will equally come from the data not performing in the way the researcher hoped, or not standing out, or not revealing anything new.

What exactly did the researcher mean by the 'yin and yang' thing and how is it that the procedure or producing an image can be both so technical yet also so apparently interpretative? In a typically convoluted piece of writing, Lacan, following Simmel's notion of interactive seeing (1921), discusses the notion of the compelling gaze and argues that it is suggestive of moments of being transfixed with an intense focus. In such moments there is something apparently reciprocal in the relationship even if one is merely gazing at an object rather than another person (Lacan 1994) – in contrast to the casual glance, the gaze 'arrests the flux of phenomena' (Bryson 1990). This, then, suggests something of the contradictory assumptions held about seeing; that it can both be said to be a process emanating from the actor to the object, yet also can be conceptualised as an equivalent process of the object making itself apparent to the actor. It is clear that the act of seeing involves a multitude of processes, decisions and interpretations, and that in at least some of these, the object is to some degree an actor in it all. Putting it another way, it is as though on certain occasions we experience the world that we see as dynamically informing us, communicating to us how it should be regarded. In light of this, and perhaps contrary even to how these medical scientists tend to describe their activity, this process of the object 'pushing back' can be seen to be incorporated in their daily practice as an important process that leads to what they eventually consider true and accurate representations.

I want to go back to the idea of drawing, which the surgeon implied when likening his scalpel to a pencil at the beginning of this chapter, to try and clarify what was alluded to in the reference to 'yin and yang', which suggests moments in which the object in question has some role in the production of the final image that is settled upon. Drawing encompasses both the idea that it is an act of removing or extracting, and the idea that it is about augmenting or amalgamating. It perhaps encapsulates what the neuroscientists meant because it is both a process of finding structures, regions, areas and of allowing them to reveal themselves. Just like lines that may have been rubbed out, or gone over repeatedly, that in combination settle at some point in a drawing, so the medical imagers constantly flip between acts of comparing, trying variants out, deleting or superimposing. The researchers spend many hours in front of their screens, trying things out, applying new filters and logarithms to the data, comparing the images they generate with atlases and other images – each time adopting mini-hypotheses about what may happen and why, and little by little constructing a dialogue between how they expect the image to look and how, at each version, it presents itself to them.

I was shown how an imager, who patiently decided to show me how she was gradually arriving at a particular scan of the bran, does this once. 'OK this is ... You know you take the coordinates. OK minus 22 so you go to minus 22. It's like map reading... You go to minus 22 ... But minus 22 doesn't exist because it was done every 4 millimetres', the junior scientist patiently explained, as her eyes continually flitted from the screen, to a book, to a chart – and to my quite clearly vacant expression. She went on, 'OK so let's say I take minus 24 ... But because I'm not very good at anatomy I use this stupid thing', and she promptly traces the coordinate using an acetate with a line drawn on. It suddenly didn't seem very scientific to an outsider like myself. 'Let's see, zero is here and minus 76 ... So you go zero here and you go minus 76 ... OK that's the cerebellum, here look, it's showing itself really clearly... So that's fine because it's a huge structure in the brain – that's the huge blob here and that's actually not very specialised …' With that, she tapped the keyboard of the computer, and the image seemed to radically change as the navigation seemed to allow her to change the image, and it shifted both in scale and plane. 'But when you look at areas that are really well functionalised like all these little differences between the medial pre-frontal cortex, the superior frontal cortex, the middle … I mean what about if this guy had a little tiny brain and it's longer or smaller?' She looks at me with an expression of exasperation, but I'm not certain whether it's because it is apparent I hadn't really been following, or if it is because she felt that she might have just demonstrated to herself once again the uncertainty and evident hesitancy of her own procedures.

Given what appears as an inherent ambiguity in daily practice, in stark contrast to the clinical precision portrayed of this incredibly advanced technology, I rather provocatively asked another junior imager if they weren't just in some way playing around, in a pretty unscientific way that contrasted with the rigid and careful procedures adopted at the beginning. 'I suppose it may seem like that,' she replied somewhat defensively, 'and it's true that there is a kind of art to this as well as a science. But we can't just do anything, you know, there are strict guidelines to everything I'm doing and trying out. It's hard … and time consuming – it's not "play" at all!' Nevertheless, to an outsider, the continuous ways in which images are produced, amended and revised, appears remarkably as though they are being manipulated according to few explicit rules. The researchers are freely able to adopt a trial and error approach to the manipulation of the data and the generation of the images. And despite the quiet environment, free of patients and the usual mess of medical practice, the main sounds to be heard and actions to be seen are the continual tapping on keyboards and shifting of computer mice, perhaps a little reminiscent of a games arcade.

By such a term as 'play', I did not mean to trivialise or undermine the activity, but instead suggest that the processes involve a dynamic interaction between trying to find or generate an image that best fits what is being expected, and discovering an image that in some sense tells its own story. Nevertheless, the very fact that certain images are settled upon, and are chosen either as best exemplars or as the basis for further research, ensures that at some point in the on-going process a particular image, and the various values and expectations that lead not simply to their production, but their selection, become fixed. To this end, and to try and piece together how the idea of drawing and playing might actually come together in the production of a specific scan, I asked a few of the junior scientists during a coffee break how they ever actually settled on one image or another. As a group they were amused by my asking, not because it didn't resonate with them, but because many felt that they weren't entirely sure either. One of them decided to speak for them all and told me, in a confessional tone, that indeed much of what they did was post hoc, and that yes, they were actively trying to make sure the scan showed what they wanted it to show, but that 'it is still science – we never make anything up.'

The glass of the monitor offers a curious but significant illusion to contain these activities. It serves to confirm a sense of transparency, and that somehow it is merely a window through which the internal body is revealed. During the trials and changes of data manipulation and the various versions of images generated, this illusion is perhaps distant, as it is evident that the appropriate or best image hasn't been settled upon. Notes are often stuck to the screen, printouts of data might lie under cold mugs of half-drunk coffee, while old images lie scattered on the desks. But the finalisation of a particular image tends to be marked by a rapid clearing away of this debris, such that its final uncluttered framing on the screen marks the very fixed nature of the image. At these times, therefore, the distance between the observer and the body, possibly scanned long ago and in another part of the building, collapses when, at last, a definite sense of something is finally observed. Other people may be invited over to comment and hopefully admire the final version, confirming its significance still further. And so the signs of labour, of the time taken to arrive at the final unambiguous picture that shows what was intended, are often discarded, leaving only the fiction of a single image, as though it had just simultaneously, and straightforwardly, appeared.

Seeing Wholes and Parts

As an observer of these observers, what is most notable in the labs where this processing work is done is the general silence of activity. Many of the researchers spend hours in front of monitors, headphones on, listening to the radio or their own choice of music. One could easily be forgiven for assuming, therefore, that the identification of significant regions or parts of an image and the final interpretation and construction of the image really was a sole pursuit, and one that simply requires dogged labour and the acquisition of individualised expert vision. Yet, in truth, conversations – though not frequent – do occur during the course of a day about the images, and what they should be doing with them. Though not visible in the final images, and the stories told about them, these fleeting exchanges allow individuals to ask each other what they make of the developing image, to confirm expectations about what might be shown, and to decide what aspects of the data might be jettisoned as extraneous complications.

Amman and Knorr-Cetina describe how, amongst a group of geneticists, verbal exchanges served to 'fix' what the scientists were examining into a stable point of reference with which to build up factual claims (Amman and Knorr-Cetina 1990). Though these informal exchanges at the lab bench would never be logged, their role was crucial, converting data into 'evidence'. A very similar process can be seen amongst the junior neuroscientists; every so often headphones are peeled back, or coffees shared, as hesitations are raised between them, while pens are tapped on the screen, or sections scrawled over on printouts, as they chat and discuss what the image is actually showing. Thus, the apparent individual nature of the process, and the silence that symbolises it, is just occasionally disrupted: 'What do you make of this bit here? Clearly the insulas, left and right ... as well as the thalamus but what about this bit here?' said one researcher. 'I think that you have to see whether the hippocampus is really valid or something as well', came the reply. 'Yes, mmm, I think so to. But I have to be careful not to lose it.' Both stare at the screen as various options are chosen to try and ensure that various things are clearly differentiated in the image. There's a sense of frustration, as a particular part of the image resolutely appears to resist attempts to exclude it. After a few attempts, each time reverting – as far as I could make out – to the original image, the colleague shrugs his shoulders, and announces, 'Sure, but it's clearly trying to tell you something!'

The conversation continues, with both of them trying out names of specific regions that appear to be indicated in the scan and that might perhaps offer anchor points about which the final image might be generated. The shared pen taps, mutual nods and specific suggestions all serve to identify those elements that can be taken as given, and 'fix' them as the key points of reference. It is these moments of collective agreement and identification that provide the conceptual coordinates for further elaboration and exploration of the visual image itself. However, the fixing does not stop there, with mutual verbal agreements, but, since the data is so flexible, it gets folded over and hidden from view as a revised version of the scan is eventually generated. So it is that the collective language, by which the imagers effectively 'feel' their way through the dynamics of agreement and dispute in conversation, gets lost and only incorporated as something that is individual and tacit.

What these regular moments also demonstrate is the extent to which the technology continues to allow for mutual interpretations, decision making and evaluations emerging from the social, rather than strictly technical, nature of their work. Though based on highly advanced physicals and complex mathematical algorithms, the final settling of an image nevertheless requires interpretations and decisions. As we have seen, the technology does not, as might be assumed, simply generate images automatically, but in fact is so complex and the amount of data so great, that it requires a high degree of intervention by individuals and sometimes by groups of experts. In so doing, the hierarchy between senior and apprentice remains, even if the nature of the skill is tied to new areas of decision making and manipulation. It is these small interactions that suggest that the idea of drawing and playing is far more than metaphorical, but involves the interactions not merely between the objective observer and the subject being looked at, but of the expert community as a whole actively involved in orientating itself towards certain images as being legitimate and meaningful. In this way, the very opening up of the object under scrutiny involves conversations between people that allows not only for differences of opinion, but for ways of talking that necessarily invite something of the image to make its own case known. So, people will not only ask mundane invitations directed to each other, but crucially commonly configure this in terms of questions that present the image as a third party. For example, 'Well, what do you think it shows?', 'Is that bit really what I think it is?' or, 'Do you really think that I should be concentrating on this area which appears to be a robust?' The point is that though it may well be individual aspects of the image that are ostensibly discussed – specific points, or parts of the body – it is the overall scan, and principles by which it can be established upon, that are being explored through the interactions with others. What is being discussed is not really what can be seen, but what are the principles that would allow these specific things to be taken as being observable in the first place. In this performative way, both the very social nature of gaining expertise, and the invocation of the agency of the thing being viewed jointly arise. Yet, the very fact that they are almost secretive exchanges suggests that for the junior researchers, this potentially collapses the truth of what they are doing, for it invites a different order to the logic that they must first know, in order to see.

Experienced imagers are more relaxed with this apparently open process, in contrast with the junior researchers who frequently flounder around, spending many weeks trying to establish what they consider to be a definitive, accurate objective image. For the more senior staff, the scientific integrity is not under threat in the multitude of processes and decisions that occur between collecting the data and representing it; one said: 'This is cutting edge research that we're doing – each scan is both compared to a normal brain, and is used to further our knowledge of the averaged brain – so there's always a great to-ing and fro-ing in our work – and that's what makes it so compelling.' 'Some have actually called it intuition,' said one of the neuroscientists, chuckling, to me, 'but it's more that I just know what to look for – not in the detail of every little speck and dot, but in the relationship between structures. It takes years of practice, and staring at these things, to have a sense of what should be where, and when it's not.'

In this simple exegesis of expert confidence, we once again see something of the tension that I have been alluding to throughout this chapter: that the scientist sees by drawing; that is, that both a model of the expected representation and the actual image are brought together in relationship. The scientist himself clearly does not feel that the process is simply a matter of comparison, but is more dialogical, in that it concerns the relationships between lines and entities in the image, rather than simply being a matter of transposing one upon the other. This Gestalt-like hypothesis is attractive, in that it stresses the underlying relationality of the details, such that they are only interpreted as meaningful because of their context. All this certainly endorses something of a mystique around expert vision – one in which learning to see is an individual process acquired by experience and studious dedication. And, in the context of what is assumed to be one of the most technical and procedural methods of medical imaging, what is striking is the way in which this value in the interpretative basis of medicine is not merely contained, but placed at the centre of a definition of expertise.

Concluding Remarks

As one junior researcher, ambitious to become a leading neuroscientist, said: 'I mean, you can only work on the question you have asked ... it's very specific. The way we analyse data is supposed to answer this question, the way you write results and generate an image, you are normally only allowed to talk about your question, not other questions you didn't ask at the beginning... so most of the time I'm trying my best not to start another story... But err, well in truth, probably, well, Seniors do do that.' I have sketched how the imager's role is to ensure data that are relevant, legitimately filtered and cleansed, such that a strikingly clear image is obtained. In order to do so it is necessary to establish, from quite an early stage in the scan production, a set of key notions and expectations from which the architecture of the final image can be gradually built. In essence, there is a kind of reverse engineering that accompanies the usual linearity of the experiment. At the centre of this two-way conjuncture in the development of the image is a skill in which the scans arise from a dual direction, something I have here referred to as drawing. The point is that seeing and knowing are not two distinct operations that can be understood according to either one pre-empting the other. Rather, the practice of the imagers in the lab, like the surgeon, is a combined process of confirming expectations and revealing variation. What is significant, however, is the way in which this combined process is never conveyed, and the way in which an idea of skill is itself implicitly used not merely to endorse ideas of professional expertise, but also to ensure that the narrative of knowing and seeing can be constructed.

Though the senior imagers have forgotten how this was acquired, assuming it to be an individually learnt process acquired through hours and hours of solitary graft, the momentary interruptions amongst more junior researchers reveal that this dialogical nature of expert vision may well be derived, quite literally, from the actual snippets of dialogue exchanged in the lab. Skill is therefore suggestive of a number of different ways in which decisions and awareness are acquired; it is as much embodied and unconscious as conscious and deliberate. But my emphasis has also been on how accounts from both surgeons and the neuroscientists suggest that this intangible nature actually serves as the means by which status is attested, and how it shapes the interactions between senior and junior staff. Because of the sense that what is acquired has a multiple nature, there is an inherent contradiction in the idea of scientific or medical education, which in their explicit forms only ever emphasise the rational, consciously and frequently rote internalisation of units of facts. In both procedures, of the scalpel or computer keyboard, there is a continual oscillation between decisions and procedures thought to 'reveal', 'unmask' or clarify structures and regions, and others that actively seek and pursue them, catching sight of them in the chaos and complexity of the data. Here, then, there is the backwards and forwards movement that the idea of drawing, and playing with drawing, encompasses. The final image may have a sense of penetrating closeness, yet its production is far less fixed.

At the heart of this dynamic, and one that perhaps explains the way in which seeing can at times be redefined as a gaze, is one of the very principles of modernity that Latour questions: the secure divide that is assumed between subject and object (Latour 1993). Medical professionals may well attempt to endorse this division much of the time, but at key moments it is as though the very subjectivity of the object, perhaps emanating from the realisation that these objects are in fact parts of people, shouts for recognition. 'The problem, as I see it, is not with the technology in terms of "Do we have the right resolution?" or "Do we have the right equipment?", but it's with things like "Are we asking the right questions?" and "Are we averaging, and fractionating in the right way?" and "Do the images reveal what we want?".' Both the junior surgeon and the junior neuroscientists appear a little uncomfortable with conceding this, in that it is felt to be a very unscientific acknowledgement. It also potentially undermines the investment they have in their eventual acquisition of expertise. But what is striking is the ease with which senior people in both fields of medicine are so relaxed with the idea that their status lies in allowing such a distinction to be temporarily, at least, blurred; that they needn't pretend that either knowing or seeing necessarily precede each other.

References

Amman, K. and K. Knorr-Cetina, 1990. 'The Fixation of (Visual) Evidence,' in *Representation in Scientific Practice*, eds. M. Lynch and S. Woolgar. London and Cambridge, Mass.: MIT Press.

Bal, M. 2003. 'Visual Essentialism and the Object of Visual Culture', *Journal of Visual Culture* 2 (1): 5–32.

Benjamin, W. 1999 'The Work of Art in the Age of Mechanical Reproduction', in *Illuminations*. London: Pimlico.

Blume, S. 1992. *Insight and Industry: Technological Change in Medicine*. Cambridge: Cambridge University Press.

Bryson, N. 1990. *Looking at the Overlooked: Four Essays on Still Life Painting*. London: Reaktion.

Bynum, W.F. and R. Porter. 1993. 'The Art and Science of Medicine', *Companion Encyclopedia of the History of Medicine*, eds. W.F. Bynum and R. Porter. London and New York: Routledge.

Classen, C. 1997. 'Foundations for an Anthropology of the Senses', *UNESCO* 153: 401–12.

Hacking, I. 1999. *The Social Construction of What?* Cambridge, Mass. and London: Harvard University Press.

Ingold, T. 2000. *The Perception of the Environment: Essays in Livelihood, Dwelling and Skill*, Chapter 13: 'The Journey along a Way of Life: Maps, Wayfinding and Navigation'. London and New York: Routledge.

Jay, M. 1992. 'Scopic Regimes of Modernity', in *Modernity and Identity*, eds. S. Lash and J. Friedman. Oxford: Blackwell.

Jenks, C., ed. 1995. Introduction, 'The centrality of the eye in Western culture', in *Visual Culture.* London and New York: Routledge.

Kember, S. 1998. *Virtual Anxiety: Photography, New Technologies and Subjectivity.* Manchester: Manchester University Press.

Kevles, B.H. 1997. *Naked to the Bone: Medical Imaging in the Twentieth Century.* Reading, Mass.: Addison-Wesley.

Lacan, J. 1994. *The Four Fundamental Concepts of Psycho-analysis.* Harmondsworth: Penguin Books.

Latour, B. 1993. *We Have Never Been Modern.* New York: Harvester Wheatsheaf.

Lynch, M. and S. Woolgar, eds. 1990. *Representation in Scientific Practice.* Cambridge, Mass.: MIT Press.

Rousseau, J-J. 1969. *Emile.* London: Dent.

Simmel, G. 1921. 'Sociology of the Senses: Visual Interaction', in *Introduction to the Science of Sociology*, eds. R. Park and E. Burgess. Chicago: University of Chicago Press.

Chapter 5

Learning within the Workplaces of Artists, Anthropologists and Architects: Making Stories for Drawings and Writings

Wendy Gunn

Introduction

Anthropology can contribute to an understanding of everyday working practices of artists, anthropologists and architects by situating both knowledge and skills within their social context. Artists', anthropologists' and architects' working processes should be understood not as a series of abstract actions, carried on in isolation from the social world, but rather as the activity of persons situated within a field of social relations. This challenges assumptions that an interior process of thought controls action, and that thinking is separate from doing. I consider here the difference, and the relation, between direct and indirect forms of communication within fine art, anthropological and architectural design practice. Referring to ethnographic materials from fieldwork in artists' and architects' workplaces and reflections on my own practices as an anthropologist, I ask how learning within a situated context is mediated by stories and/or drawing and imaging skills.

By placing artists', architects' and anthropologists' drawings and writings within a network of sociotechnical relations, I challenge normative historical models of fine art, anthropological and architectural practice that position drawing, imaging and writing skills outside of the actualities of the everyday. The problem is to discover how these representations are integrated into the course of situated actions within specific environmental contexts. As a means of comparing art, anthropological and architectural knowledge traditions, I question how skilled practitioners learn and how memory, like the body to which it belongs, undergoes continual generation and regeneration in the contexts of an individual's life activities within an environment. Placing analysis of institutional modes of learning across the disciplines of fine art, anthropology and architecture alongside narratives of learning within the workplaces and field sites of artists, anthropologists and architects, I aim to show how information transmitted through formal instruction relates to the skills that learners develop through their own practical experiments.

I have extensive experience of fine art education and practice, architectural teaching and collaborative architectural practice alongside research training in social anthropology. This background was essential in negotiating a middle ground between my informants and myself as an anthropologist. Such an ambiguous position allowed me to mediate and remain responsive to situations as they unfolded (Gunn 2002: 31). My doctoral research in social anthropology was concerned with architectural knowledge and changing technologies of contemporary architectural practice. The thesis argument focused on the relations between agents and technologies and on the representation of those relations, working between the realms of the abstract and the material. Developing this research within the context of an art school (2002–2005), I am examining the ways in which storytelling, drawing, imaging and writing mediate the processes of situated learning. Specifically, I am concerned with how speech, gesture, graphic expression and written words all work together in specific contexts of interaction, highlighting both the coupling of perception and action and the role of narrative in artists' and teachers' working practices. Extending my research beyond the art school context, I compare how artists, architects and anthropologists engage with their sites of practice. Focusing on the interrelations between perception, creativity and skill, I look at the ways in which their work shapes and is shaped by their engagements with land and landscape, and how these engagements might be translated into contexts of learning.

Taking as my starting point Leroi Gourhan's notion that intelligence lies in human gesture itself, as a synergy of human being, tool and raw material, it becomes apparent that the interrelationships between perception, creativity and skill are fundamental while studying how a person undergoes growth and development within an environment that is continually changing. How an individual perceives the environment and how this perception informs a way of being in the world raises the following questions: What does it mean to perceive an individual as moving and actively engaging within an environment that is unfolding? And within such a context what role might the artist, anthropologist or architect play?

The journey I have attempted to develop for the reader evokes a situated practice as experienced by an artist, an anthropologist and an architect. Relations between things are far from being made explicit, for they are always in the process of becoming. Within this context, knowing, for a creative practitioner, comes from glimpses of meaning along the way, rather than being fully set out in advance of the journey (Gunn 2002: 32).

Seeing as a Way of Knowing

> Translation must always be the re-creation of the original into something profoundly different. On the other hand, it is never a substitution of word for word but invariably the translation of whole contexts. (Malinowski 1935: 11–12)

Within a creative process, movements between knowledge places distinguish the novice from the skilled practitioner. For the skilled practitioner, making is not so much about imposing as relating to or engaging with the constituents of an environment in a particular way. Thus, meanings are discovered, coming out of this particular kind of engagement, and places come into being through being involved with the activity itself. This approach differs from one that takes meaning to be overlaid upon the physical world, as if it were possible to take yourself out of it, and to place yourself above its surface.

As an anthropologist, I have been working alongside generalists, art historians, architects, artists, students and teachers as part of a larger interdisciplinary project, *Learning Is Understanding in Practice: Exploring the Interrelations between Perception, Creativity and Skill.*[1] The research project combines approaches from art and anthropology to examine the interrelations between perception, creativity and skill, through a study of the knowledge practices of fine art. The research explores the potential of a practice-based approach to teaching and learning. Central to this is the idea that learning, as exploratory practice, is itself a form of research that generates new knowledge and understanding. The project aimed to break down the divide between teaching (as the communication of pre-existing knowledge) and research (as its application) and between theory and practice. Considering connections between the disciplines of art, anthropology and architecture, skills of engaging with social and environmental conditions of site are central to my enquiry.

Interdisciplinary methods were developed in collaboration with Ingold (2003–2004) for the study of artists' and architects' skills/knowledge, involving ethnographic techniques of participant observation and hands-on learning, provided insights concerning the generation of ideas. Importantly, methodologies adopted within the field sites described were designed to connect research questions with the ethnographic practice of participant observation. The way to understand how knowledge is acquired, we contend, is for the researcher to participate in the processes of its acquisition, and to reflect critically on these from the perspective of an insider. This is fundamental to an anthropological approach adopted by the research. It is for this reason too that the research is intrinsically interdisciplinary. Moreover, our experiments in teaching and learning have contributed to our research aims of testing whether learning can be a way of doing research, and practice a way of doing theory. Comparing fine art and architectural knowledge traditions within situated contexts of learning, I reflect on my own ambiguous position as an anthropologist and what it means to draw and redraw a cut as a way of learning through doing.

My approach considers both the workplace and institutions of learning as contexts to study the interrelations, in practice, between perception, creativity and skill. I examine how creative practitioners move between a variety of materials and technologies in the exploration of innovative practices. Through this, I aim to understand how skills and knowledge originating from site are given value. I focus on learning bodily skills as a social process, which is continually responsive to others' movements. Stressing the dynamics of development leads to a focus on issues of embodiment, on the incorporation of an individual's creative capacities as he or she is continually growing. I argue that some forms of knowledge afforded within creative practice resist commodification and institutionalisation.

Skills of Engagement

> From the cycle of growth and decay
> I borrow a part and prime it;
> A simple idea applied to the qualities and circumstances of each time and place.
> (Nash, n.d.)

Had he been living in the nineteenth century the environmental sculptor David Nash[2] would have been a landscape painter. Alongside his contemporaries, Richard Long, Hamish Fulton and Roger Ackling, he wanted to find a way of being within the landscape as opposed to viewing it from a distance. David plants, prunes, grafts, trains, cultivates and cuts; he works with living and dead wood. Whilst within the landscape substance comes through growth. A tree is coming into being or going back into the earth. This is a complementary action. The living tree breathes through the seasons. Wood suits Nash's 'nature'. His interest in the process of how wood ages is reflected in his interest in how living beings undergo transformations in time. The growth of a tree, its roots, in many ways parallels an artist's development. If they have the right circumstances they will continue from their roots.

David could draw very well when he was a child. As a result of receiving praise from his family for making 'good' watercolour drawings, he continued to perfect a repertory of graphic techniques (*Nash*).[3] Years later, while developing a sculptural practice, he became dissatisfied with his mark-making capabilities. He spent two years drawing the slate tips and wooded areas surrounding his home in Blaenau Ffestiniog, trying to find appropriate 'marks of a place' to suggest a human presence in his work. Learning to extend the range of one's marks demands self-discipline and training. As a way of reworking, upgrading and fine-tuning his drawing skills, he would walk within the landscape until he found a 'subject'. Usually a relationship with land develops slowly. By thinking and feeling he made quick drawings, finding appropriate marks and materials from being outside. He returned to his studio, not with a picture but with a grasp of gestures, transferring onto paper experiences of how a line began and ended. The exercise was perceived as learning marks belonging to a place.

Drawing outside is different from drawing inside a studio. While drawing outside facts from a site speak as ideas and possibilities. Returning from his daily drawing practice outside, he said, 'his eyes were alive'. Learning to draw in this way, he said, he had experienced 'seeing'. The practice of drawing enabled him to 'adjust his attitude' towards looking more deeply at everyday environments (*Nash*). Each drawing was described as a journey. The means, duration and destination varied as much as the diversity of human beings he encountered on his travels. 'To capture meaning' an artist needs to respond to an idea, notion or feeling quickly (*Nash*). Without action a fleeting moment is lost. Drawing is this activity and often the action is short in duration and can seem complete in itself. It is important to mention that David not only draws with pencils, charcoal, pastels, wax, dirt and watercolour, he also draws with chain saws. With chain saws of different sizes he can make wooden sculptures in one fluid gesture (Nash and Daniel-McElroy 2004: 44).

As mentioned previously, David is interested in how different types of wood transform with time. Documenting processes of cracking and warping, drying and shrinking in both living and dead wood, with a camera, led him to conceive of his role, not so much as a sculptor, but as an observer. Observational skills seen alongside the social skills of listening and telling stories were fundamental in understanding site. However, as he reminded me, different kinds of stories come from making inside and outside.

Making sculpture is a practical activity and the site determines how a sculpture develops. A site has both fixed and temporal aspects and affords possibilities to apply a loose and tight relationship: loose, in the way a site is characterised by its changing time and rhythm, tight, in the sense that facts of a site remain static. Deliberating over the relation between site and place, I asked David if site and place co-existed. He replied by referring to his own experiences of being in one place for an extended period of time. Place becomes part of him and the work becomes part of place. Recalling an earlier experience when I worked with him in the northeast of Scotland,[4] David told me places are full of facts and facts are full of ideas. What emerges, comes out of what was possible at that time. As facts come, ideas emerge – importantly, I must remember I do not have to compromise ideas because facts are of a place.

Sharing and giving his artworks with and to others was an important aspect of his work as an artist. When a sculpture goes off to a gallery or private collector it becomes 'placed' or 'homed'. Very rarely does David see it again. If a sculpture is returned to the studio after a public exhibition he feels it has been given value, a wealth has returned to the object. The movement outwards has reawakened a sculpture's potential because the wood has came back with a history of being experienced by others. At the start of a project he has learned to name and address each new person he is working with. Working with wood is very similar. It may not appear necessary to know the name of the tree but it is essential when making a cut – what is this material like? Meeting wood is a physical activity and the feeling of making is in the wood and can be experienced by others. It is important therefore to get rid of anxiety and observe yourself while working with the material. For David, involving others in the physical activity of making a wooden sculpture is the most fulfilling way of engaging with a site.

Figure 5.1 shows a photograph of a working drawing explaining to others the actions required to carve a pyramid, sphere and cube out of wood. According to David, the chalk marks inscribed on the surface of a tree trunk say everything about what he is as a person. He is 'materials, measuring instruments, tools and the human me'. When I asked him what he learned from working with wood he said, 'There is this body of knowledge. This body is in my body' (*Nash*).

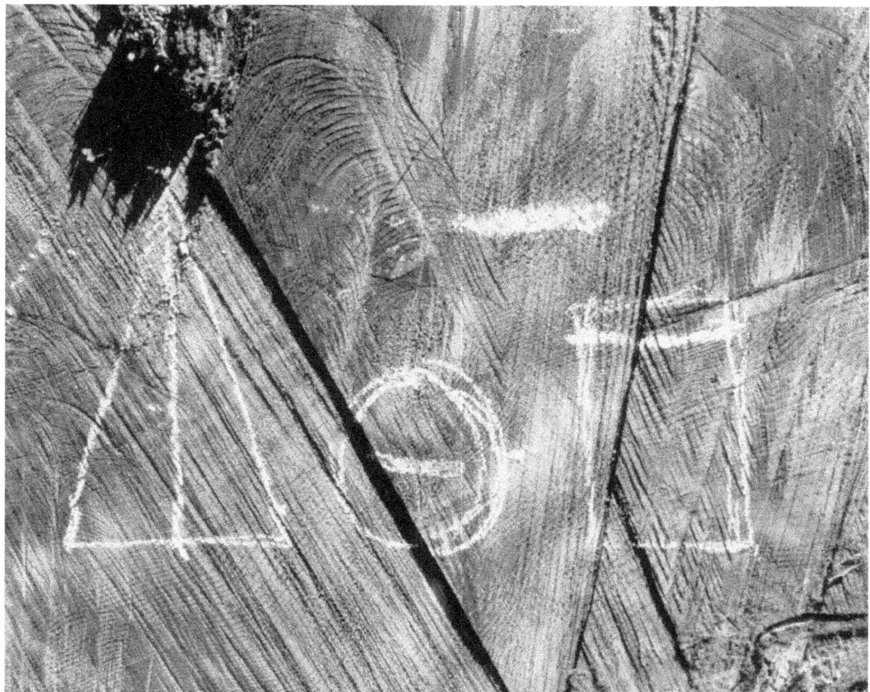

Figure 5.1'*Pyramid, sphere and cube' (2003), a photograph by David Nash.* (All rights reserved)

Drawing and Redrawing the Line of a Cut

While trying to understand artists' skills within situated contexts of learning, I set myself the task of drawing David's cuts in wood and redrawing his drawings of such cuts. He recommended that I begin drawing trees and branches (outside) to understand movement. Cut lines in David's sculptures are meant to be angular and geometric in form. Geometry represents an order in nature, a path – like the line of a cut. He said, 'It is the poetry and geometry of movement that interests me. When we think of geometry, we don't think of movement' (Nash 2004: 49). Movement, according to David, is not only a practical necessity in making sculpture; it is essential for generating ideas by chance.

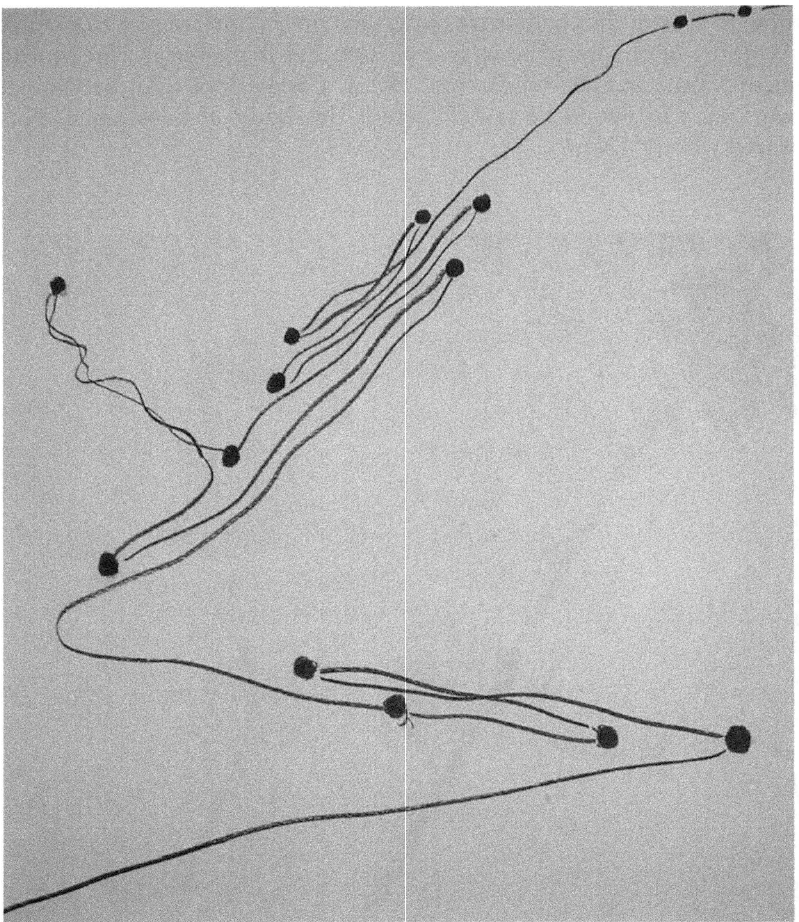

Figure 5.2 *'Journey line' (2004), a drawing by David Nash.* (All rights reserved)

In order to understand the similarities and differences between working outside and inside a studio space, I spent time moving between different places of making within David's working environments: Capel Rhiw (a former Calvinist/ Methodist chapel which functions as a sculpture studio and archive), Coen-y-coed (a woodland area and place for growing sculptural works) and his drawing studio. Within these learning contexts I worked between the media of drawing, writing and photography, trying to understand a creative process, which left wood in a 'rough state, showing the mark of the tool' (*Nash*). Drawing between inside and outside environments made me aware of cuts, cracks and splits in wood revealing and defining internal and external spaces, whereas my field notes describing how the sculptural pieces were constructed helped in attending to David's methods of attaching, fastening, joining and binding wood. Trying to find ways of describing the relations between his sculptures in Capel Rhiw, while sculptures were continually coming and going, I developed a set of questions related to the specificity of his practice for our evening discussions.

Working within the drawing studio, I discovered that 50 percent cotton paper holds and suspends charcoal dust thus creating depth. The blackness achieved communicated both an absence and presence of a cut in wood. Attempting to copy this process while redrawing David's later wooden boulder drawings (Figure 5.2).[5] I realised that the strength of his marks was dependent on an ability to absorb errors into drawings. I also became aware that making the drawings was not just a matter of joining dots with a line. The line was not continuous and the gestural flow was interrupted by black charcoal dust rubbings, implying a time, place and story. Whereas my task was identifying the problems with trying to imitate David's working practices, David had to find ways of demystifying rather than obscuring his concepts for other people. Common to us both was an interest in making an object capable of transcending the boundaries between ways of working and knowing specific to the disciplines of art and anthropology.

It is difficult to redraw a drawing, especially when someone who has been making gestural responses towards an environment and documenting his activities for thirty-seven years has made the lines. Even David has difficulty producing the same line for editions of drawings commissioned by galleries. He has found each time he redraws the line it is different. I suggest it is this slightness of difference in mark-making, achieved through a process of reproduction and innovation, that inspires his drawing practice.

It is in the Telling

Within an architectural working process there are different ways of drawing. There are also many different ways of thinking about how drawings can be involved in a process of communication which is both multi-disciplinary and collaborative. Architects involve drawings on many levels of their work, moving between different drawing tools and surfaces, depending on the preference and skills of the architect and the project involved.

Knut-Eirik Dahl is an architect and former partner in the internationally recognised architectural practice Blå Strek Architects (1982–92). Since 1992, Dahl has been director of Dahl Architects, located in Tromsø, Norway. His practice concentrates on large-scale urban design proposals, competitions and housing projects. I lived for twelve months in Tromsø (1998–99), during which time I conducted formal interviews with the architect concerning the relations between his practices of describing, systems of notation and the impact of incorporating computer-aided design (CAD) tools into the design process. Knut-Eirik speaks of the act of drawing as a kind of performance, where he works in many rooms drawing on a series of boards. He said, 'It is like creating a kind of theatre where everything is possible' (*Dahl*). Somehow, I could never imagine him being content sitting in front of a computer for many hours producing CAD-generated drawings. The few drawings that he has managed to produce, while developing his urban design proposals, originate from listening to and learning from voices in the city that have something to say. They were described by Knut-Eirik as drawings of discussions. Although drawing was an extension of language and language is understood as being connected to personhood, his way of being a person was more important than his way of drawing (*Dahl*). He felt that working at a slow pace is essential if one is to discover new concepts while making a visual image. It is equally essential if one is to represent, in the abstract, a concept that already exists but which has no material counterpart in the visible geography of the site. Working with a watercolour collage during the development of a design or concept enables Knut-Eirik to work at a slow pace. In his collage, the tunnels and roads took second place to a new form of organisation that requires slower movement. Through this mode of representation he presented his critical view of the organisation of the city around mechanical speed. At the same time, increased mechanical speed interested Knut-Eirik because of its capacity to compress an unknown landscape, rendering it more accessible to small existing communities (*Dahl*).

In executing his watercolours Knut-Eirik combines layer upon layer of transparent wash with fine black ink on the paper surface. Describing the technique, he remarked:

> You may not have a thought in your head but when you touch paper, something comes out of it. So it is my body actually and I have an extra mind, an extra body and an extra weapon that no one else has, and it is drawing in the way that I do. (*Dahl*)

Adding layer upon layer leads to the discovery of the latent possibilities in the landscape and in nature. For Knut-Eirik the watercolour collage is a way of developing a concept and is more important to him than detailed construction drawings. It becomes a way of studying his own interactions within a mirrored landscape, which operates at a slow speed and in slow motion. 'Sometimes,' he says, 'I can forget everything and drown myself in drawing' (*Dahl*). The space of his office was for him a free space where the mind could move more slowly, and where long periods of time were spent finding new ways to think. Knut-Eirik's way of working was not an immediate form of image making. This was deliberate and intended as a critical response to architects' preoccupation with speeding up the design process by means of CAD tools. He admired artists' understanding of tactility in their drawing and believed this tactility to be crucial to avoid the flatscapes created by the graphic quality of the architect's line.

Making watercolour drawings requires slowness, not speed. As Knut-Eirik insisted, his watercolours are not flatscapes. They have depth, and cannot be interpreted immediately. Knut-Eirik made drawings for himself, in order to see beyond the surface and be taken on a journey, revealing many landscapes within the transparent washes of colour. Knowledge learned through these journeys opens up many worlds. Ingold, similarly, describes a narrative journey as one where the act of telling a story allows both the teller and the listener to become immersed in a world that has transparency and depth, 'transparency, because one can see into it; depth, because the more one looks the further one sees' (Ingold 2000: 56). And as Jackson argues, it is by making explicit the relations between discourse and practice through the structure of the narrative, that it connects with the everyday (Jackson 1996: 39).

The Writing, the Telling and the Discussions

Knut-Eirik knew that very few people understood his drawings. They were a way of communicating with himself. Since they were never intended as a means of explaining his ideas to others, he had to spend much time elaborating his ideas in discussion (Meløe 1983: 91). A different type of drawing, which he regarded as a kind of 'primitive drawing', was made for clients, consultants and the public (*Dahl*). Knut-Eirik always saw drawings as part of a text, and the images he found in his own writings, and in the writings of others, were for him a source of inspiration during the formative development of an architectural design. He understood the text as helping him to discover something that is known. Taken together, Knut-Eirik considered drawing and texts as kinds of story, closer to fiction. In his work, writing was seen to be just as important as speaking and was never intended to describe a final project. He made no distinction between drawing and writing and did not consider writings or drawings to be end points in themselves. Rather, their importance lies in helping him to tell a story involving many people. Considering the role of visual images in the stories of architects, the Norwegian philosopher Jakob Meløe remarked that, 'If we think of architectural representations as visual diagrams, then stories help explain the visual diagram to other people.'[6] The act of telling a story can be likened to a narrative journey of exploration and discovery. Through getting to know a site the architect is reminded of a particular instance, landscape feature or memory of engagements with other people. Memories of a site endure long after the memory of its architecture fades. These memories provide guidance throughout the design and building process in a way that is not so much about physical orientation as about value judgements.

Stories told verbally are different from lecture notes belonging to architects. Written words have to be specific and the writer must know in advance where he or she is going. The story, by contrast, can repeat itself – allowing listeners space to remember. It is more immediate, and can be altered depending on whether it is intended for other architects, the client or the consultant. An architect's story takes an architectural idea beyond formal geometric or geographical understanding. The design unfolds through telling stories and the story becomes intertwined with both the architect's and the project's identity. Stories are not imposed upon the world, they conduct an architect's way into it, delineating both self and the physical environment upon which she or he is focused (Gunn 2002: 91).

Conversational Aspects of Knowledge

In the context of an art school (2003–2005),[7] I worked alongside graduate students taking the Master's Fine Art programme at the University of Dundee. This involved participating in student seminars, studio critiques and lectures, as an external adviser, teacher and observer. In parallel, I attended undergraduate life-drawing classes and interviewed life-drawing teachers and models. The question I keep returning to after conducting seventeen months of fieldwork is: Why did I learn more from the processes of making within the workplaces of artists and architects than in a contemporary institution of learning?

In a fine art school the oral nature and one-to-one nature of teaching means a lot of teaching and learning is exchanged and shared but never written down. Teaching and learning occurs predominately in shared studios. Within the corridors leading to the studios one can smell paint, printmaking ink and sawn wood from the woodworking workshop. The skills taught within these contexts cannot be conveyed in an office situation, lecture theatre or seminar room. Often students are told stories by their teacher related to the teacher's own experience of making as an artist. However, most teachers I interviewed agreed that it was not enough merely to tell a student about their experiences of making and all that was necessary to know. How a story is told makes knowledge appropriate. Students have to find their own way and way-finding involves learning to pay attention to environmental features. Seeing becomes a way of knowing and learning involves feeling one's way into a situated context. The amount of time required to learn is crucial, recognising that the person who learns requires experience and opportunities to relate new knowledge in order to understand. A number of fine art teachers commented that the problem with many of the younger students is that they have learned 'to say the right things by jumping through a series of hoops'. This mode of learning unfortunately did not always lead the student to an understanding of what they were saying.

Many of the students I have been working with have difficulties in writing about their practice. Composing a text is to follow a stream of consciousness and write down whatever comes into their thoughts at a specific moment in time. Although fine art students have developed a form of critical writing based on their experiences of studio practice, writing essays, dissertations and the doctoral thesis are increasingly becoming an important means of validating both undergraduate and postgraduate studies in fine art. This has led to a greater stigma being attached to students who have problems with reading and writing than if they had a problem with their drawing. Fine art students' writing is often demanded, threatened or forced by tutors. Often the texts are read and marked by one lecturer with a background in art history, theory or critical studies, and no direct experience of practice. While recognising that a small number of students are eloquent writers and do involve writing as part of their fine art practice, many are terrified of the written word. This fear is linked to an inability to change what has been written. Frequently art students ask lecturers in history and theory why they have to express themselves in words. After all, they do not want to be writers – they want to be artists and as such are not interested in composing texts with letters, words, sentences and punctuation (*Todman*).

Speaking, Writing, Drawing and Imaging

Tangled threads originate from 'a confused knotted mess, teased out between pins into organised rope' (*Todman*). Amy's words drawn on the pages of her sketchbook are a trace – marks suggesting the process of making an installation. The words are a form of inscription and as such are not meant as a description *of* or *about* a finished object; rather they are essential *for* a process of describing a thing being made. She works with pins, matches, sticks and lines. Drawings of tangled threads keep things outside and, for the duration of making three-dimensional constructions, tangled threads gather things together. Finding a place where threads started and ended inspired Amy to write and draw in her sketchbook. Looking through her sketchbooks together she said, 'the writings are a kind of drawing' (*Todman*). Amy was a fourth-year undergraduate student in fine art when we first met in 2003 to discuss the relation between drawing and writing within her working process. Writing has always been difficult for her and she tries to find ways of avoiding it. Comparing the practice of writing with her practice of drawing she said, 'I have difficulty with writing because it separates thoughts, my ideas bring drawing and writing together.' Usually she writes and draws at the same time.

Despite Amy's anxiety with learning how to write she enjoys reading and makes books, 'even though they are picture books' (*Todman*). Words do not make Amy feel 'safe' because they make relations with friends and teachers uncomfortable. Her writing is considered 'too nice' and she has been told on numerous occasions that she is not good at writing. As a result she does not enjoy the process because it makes her feel inadequate. It is easier for others, if she makes her writings completely abstract. Writing skills involve self-discipline and rational thought; qualities Amy has been told she does not have. Instead of agonising over her lack of ability to 'get right to the heart of the matter' by writing things down, she relies on her artwork to speak for itself. Preferring speaking to writing, Amy is good at talking about her work through gesticulated movements of the body.

Sketches are 'a build-up of lines' (*Todman*) and the act of sketching involves taking dead ends, keeping on going and reflecting. Gathering drawings and writings together within the pages of a sketchbook, make patterns that help the practitioner 'feel what is going on' (*Todman*). Through this process Amy's intention is not to portray a form of reality. 'Describing' in her practice is a doing word; the acts of sketching, drawing and making can be compared to a form of poetics.[8] creating a possibility for finding her own voice. Poetics in this sense allows thought to grow and images to gather and enfold into themselves. Her tangled threads become less tangled and more easily understood after speaking with her teacher, suggesting the line that originates from direct interaction with oral narrative leads to a more open means of communication. The sketches and three-dimensional drawings make sharing and divergence in her work possible, whereas, she said, there is 'no room for her' in writing to do that.

Moments of clarity within a practice-based learning process are a private, experience, according to Jan, and are difficult to translate into words. I first saw Jan's sketchbooks in 2003 while attending her Fine Art degree exhibition at the University of Dundee. Of particular interest was a series of sketchbooks revealing detailed studies of her interactions within non-urban landscapes. As someone who entered art school training after studying geography at university, she was concerned that the visual in her work was not communicating. At first she had notebooks for writing and sketchbooks for drawing, but soon became frustrated by the need to have words and drawings in separate places. Her sketchbooks always provoked a more positive reaction in her teachers than finished artworks. For Jan sketchbooks provided places where explorations of many dimensions were allowed to happen, inspiring her to describe things not made visible before. Aware that writing still dominated her work she pointed with frustration at pages containing only texts describing her practical investigations. Jan's aim was to practically engage with ideas and not to write about doing them. Comparing notebooks recording geological field visits with sketchbooks documenting studio experiments, she said, 'describing a process is a struggle because you have a tension between describing and what is being described'. Sketchbooks are precious because they *are* direct observations, taken from source and not from memory, second-hand or someone else's experience. A sketchbook is understood as possessing a form of authenticity because the materials within it would be impossible to remember at a later point (*Hendry*). Each page reveals non-visual and visual experiences from a particular time and place. The action of sketching is a way of remembering, later reenacted during a process of making. Remembering a process of making is similar, then, to how one would remember a story or a journey, confirming Ingold's point that knowledge is integrated along a path of movement (Ingold 2005: 8). Jan's sketchbook was a place to 'watch both herself and her processes of working – in nature, recording movement through writing, scribbling and taking photographs for her book'. Within this place she was able to make partial connections between different strands of knowledge, which had become separated in her field notebooks (Strathern 1991: 53). During our conversation she turned the pages of her sketchbook, stopping at a sketch of tree branches, shown in Figure 5.3.

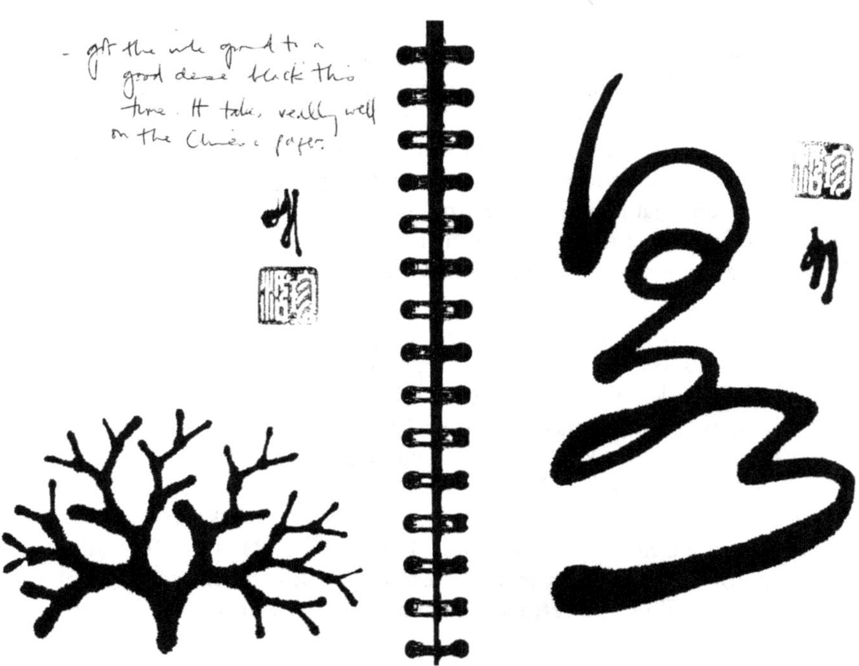

Figure 5.3 *'Thinking of tree branches …', a page from Jan's sketchbook.*

The interconnecting branches in Jan's sketches remind us of Carruthers' discussion of medieval cognitive pattern making, as a way of locating knowledge within and in relation to other things. Importantly, 'Placement and location, the "mapping" of material, are necessary to remembering and thinking' (Carruthers 1998: 34). Reflecting on her previous scientific education, Jan said the sketches of trees were a way of resisting an oversimplification of knowledge systems. It was therefore necessary to make correspondences between things through the act of sketching itself. Working in this way, her sketchbook helped to recover experiences within specific places at particular moments in time. By contrast, field notebooks contained information that was finished, and considered essential to producing an accurate report about geological findings (Goodwin 1994: 608).

Growth, Lines and Cuts

Knowing a site for David, Knut-Eirik and myself comes from direct experience of active engagement (Toren 1995: 164). Our stories of learning from a project, field and architectural site suggest that through the performative acts of making, continuity is manifested between present and past. (Toren 1995: 164, 168)

The cuts in David's wooden sculptures and the layers of wash contained within Knut-Eirik's watercolours implicate an absence and a presence in their work. In both instances, in the process of making and the objects made, depth and slowness are given value. Returning to questions I posed earlier – What does it mean to perceive an individual as moving and actively engaging within an environment that is unfolding? And within such a context, what role might the artist or architect play? – from the materials presented I propose that it is through the act of storytelling a creative practitioner is able to share and make accessible experiences of engaging with a site. Someone who can 'tell', as Ingold has argued, is attuned to picking up information in the environment that others, less skilled in the tasks of perception, might miss, and the teller, in rendering his knowledge explicit, conducts the attention of his audience along the same paths as his own (2000: 190).

Nash and Dahl are skilled at encompassing indeterminate processes while telling others, less skilled than themselves, ways into a site. This skilled practice confirms Ingold's point that a 'storyteller who knows as he goes is neither making a map nor using one' (Ingold 2000: 230–31). Instead, telling stories involving drawings is a process more akin to *mapping* than *map-making*. Each telling is a retracing of sculptures and drawings already made, while at the same time revealing threads of what is to become. Seeing, in this sense, is comparable to Weiner's description of how Foi people of Papua New Guinea understand vision: 'not a thing of surfaces but revealed interiors' (Weiner 2001: 120). In both cases the artist and architect combine and recombine 'facts' of a site with subjective forms of knowledge. Following on from Ingold's (2000) and Turnbull's (1996, 1998) discussions of the distinction between mapping and map-making, further work is required to understand how objective and subjective knowledges become intertwined as a form of resistance in situated contexts of learning.

Recognising that the body is learning from its context, translation of embodied knowledge gained through drawing and making objects is not simply a process of copying information (Bateson 1958: 286). Movement between places and from one form to another in translation is central to understanding the interrelationships between speaking, writing, drawing and imaging, in specific contexts of interaction. Amy and Jan's sketchbooks highlight the way that speaking, writing, drawing and imagings are interwoven through the performative act within situated contexts of learning. Performativity locates seeing in embodied practice and notions of place are central to locations of becoming. Within their sketchbooks the fear of writing described earlier does not exist. Each page provides a place for not knowing where their journey will take them, finding their way about because text, image, gesture and speech are integrated together. When they are lost within their practice, it is drawing and not writing that helps them find their way.

Synthesis of word and image within fine art students' sketchbooks, suggests further work is required to understand the similarities and differences between non-prescriptive and prescriptive thinking; and in so doing, tracing the shift in art school education from local, subjective and qualitative knowledge traditions towards 'the'[9] importing of analytical methods and theoretical models, common to scientific explanation, into practice-based teaching, learning and research. What this change may imply is a lack of understanding of the skills required to engage with sites of practice. Attunement towards fluctuations within an environment that is never quite the same from one moment to the next is as relevant to the practices of artists, anthropologists and architects. Somehow, as Susanne Küchler has said, it is necessary to recover this kind of engagement, evocative of the thing being made by problematising the idea of learning.[10]

The question remains within a measuring or benchmarking assessment: What happens to forms of knowledge that cannot be written down? Learning and teaching in institutions where productivity and success is dependant on an audit culture focusing on targets, outputs, accountability and standardisation of criteria upon which departments can be judged (Leach 2005: 12), is there a danger in borrowing methods and systems of representation from one form into another, considering what is of value in one knowledge tradition may not have value in another? While trying to understand why I learned more from processes of making within artists' and architects' workplaces than in a contemporary institution of learning, my research returns to the broader question of how information transmitted through formal instruction relates to skills that learners develop through their own experiments. Skill is often understood as the mere application of knowledge. This implies, however, that knowledge is transmitted in a disembodied, context-free form – that is, as information – independently and in advance of its application in specific contexts of practice. From the ethnographic materials discussed, 'skilled vision' consists in the embodied capacities of action and perception that practitioners develop throughout life in the course of their practical activities. In this sense, skill is the very ground of knowledge, and not merely its application.

Understanding processes of how artists, anthropologists and architects engage with sites of practice is as much an investigation into the growth and form of the person as it is about the objects that are made. The research presented implies that the practices of making, involving others within an environment, allows for growth in the same way as a tree 'is a story of the events that have happened to it' (*Nash*).

Acknowledgements

Discussions with David Nash, Knut-Eirik Dahl, Jacob Meløe, Tim Ingold, James Leach, Susanne Küchler, Murdo Macdonald and David Turnbull, their intellectual input and critique, was fundamental to the arguments developed in this chapter. Earlier versions of the chapter were presented to the joint Aberdeen – St. Andrews postgraduate workshop, University of Aberdeen (2004), 'Modes of Becoming' research seminar, Dundee Contemporary Arts (2004), the workshop on 'Creativity' at the Department of Social Anthropology, University of Aberdeen (2004), and the 'Skilled Visions' panel, European Association of Social Anthropologists Conference, University of Vienna, 2004. In revising it for publication, I have benefited from the advice of many people, including Cristina Grasseni and Michael Herzfeld. I am indebted to both staff and students at The School of Fine Art, Dundee University for sharing their valuable experiences of making. Thanks also to members of the Creativity and Practice Research Group working on the *Learning is Understanding in Practice* research project at the Department of Anthropology, Aberdeen University and the School of Fine Art, Dundee University. Without their collaboration a rethinking of interdisciplinary work would not be possible. I gratefully acknowledge the financial support of the Economic and Social Research Council and the Arts and Humanities Research Board for the fieldwork, and of the Arts and Humanities Research Board during the writing of the chapter.

Notes

1 See, http://www.abdn.ac.uk/creativity and practice/

2 David Nash lives and works in Blaenau Ffestiniog, North Wales. The artist is represented by the Annely Juda Fine Art, London; Galerie LeLong in Paris, Zurich and New York; Galerij S65, Aaist, Belgium; Nishimura Gallery, Tokyo and the Haines Gallery, San Francisco. He was elected a Royal Academician in 1999, the same year in which he was appointed a

Research Fellow, University of Northumbria, Newcastle and was awarded an Honorary Doctorate in Art & Design by Kingston University.

3 In this instance and hereafter, except where reference is explicitly made to published and bibliographic sources, I acknowledge material gathered from discussions with named informants. To avoid confusion between primary and secondary sources all surnames of people I have been working with, and whose words are reproduced here, are italicised.

4 I participated in the workshop on *Crafting Glass* in Lybster, Caithness (2003), which Nash directed.

5 The wooden boulder drawings documented the movement and transformation of a cut wooden boulder as it journeyed through a stream, estuary and finally out to sea (1978–2003).

6 Jakob Meløe participated in the one-day interdisciplinary workshop, *Landscape Perception and the Architectural Design Process*. The workshop, held at the University of Tromsø, Norway in 1998, was an integral part of my field investigations involving philosophers, architects, historians of craft and technology, anthropologists and doctoral research students from these disciplines. Focusing on the construction and experience of the built environment, the interdisciplinary group considered the role of designs and plans in the architectural design process, the relation between design and practice, and the conditions that promote persistence or change in the forms of activity and artefacts across generations.

7 Fieldwork was carried out at the School of Fine Art, Duncan of Jordanstone College of Art and Design, University of Dundee.

8 Herzfeld's references to the original Greek verb for action (poieõ) as an analytical approach to the uses of rhetorical form and aesthetics (poiein), focusing on the relationship between form and action, have helped clarify the meaning of poetics and aesthetics within the practices discussed (Herzfeld 1997).

9 Macdonald argues that to give 'the' direction would be to invite reductionism. To give 'a' direction recognises interdisciplinarity (Macdonald 2004).

10 A recommendation by Susanne Küchler to members of the Creativity and Practice Research Group, while developing the interdisciplinary research project, *Learning is Understanding in Practice: Exploring the Interrelations between Perception, Skill and Creativity.* Advisory board meeting, Dundee Contemporary Arts, May 2003.

References

Bateson, G. 1958. *Naven: the Culture of the Iatmul People of New Guinea as Revealed through a Study of the 'Naven' Ceremonial.* Stanford: California University Press.

Carruthers, M. 1998. *The Craft of Thought: Meditation, Rhetoric and the Making of Images, 400–1200.* Cambridge: Cambridge University Press.

Goodwin, C. 1994. 'Professional Vision', *American Anthropologist* 96 (3): 606–33.

Gunn, W. 2002. *'The Social and Environmental Impact of Incorporating Computer Aided Design Technologies into an Architectural Design Process'*. Unpublished Ph.D. dissertation. Department of Social Anthropology. University of Manchester.

Herzfeld, M. 1997. *Cultural Intimacy: Social Poetics in the Nation-State.* New York: Routledge, 142–43.

Ingold, T. 2000. *The Perception of the Environment: Essays in Livelihood, Dwelling and Skill.* London and New York: Routledge.

—— 2005. 'Up, Across and Along', in *Creativity and Practice Research Papers*, ed. W. Gunn. Dundee: Creativity and Practice Research Group.

Jackson, M. 1996. 'Introduction. Phenomenology, Radical Empiricism and Anthropological Critique', in *Things as They Are: New Directions in Phenomenological Anthropology*, ed. M. Jackson. Bloomington: Indiana University Press.

Leach, J. 2005. 'Disciplinary Specialisation and Collaborative Endeavour: Some Challenges Presented by Sci-art Projects', in *Creativity and Practice Research Papers*, ed. W. Gunn. Dundee: Creativity and Practice Research Group.

Macdonald, M. 2004. *On the Mutual Illumination of Blindspots: Towards a Proper Methodology of Interdisciplinary Research – with Particular Regard to the Practice of Fine Art.* Unpublished manuscript, University of Dundee.

Malinowski, B. 1935. *Coral Gardens and Their Magic: a Study of the Methods of Tilling the Soil and of Agricultural Rites in the Trobriand Islands,*. Vol. 2. London: George Allen & Unwin Ltd.

Meløe, J. 1983. 'The Agent and his World', in *Praxeology: an Anthology*, ed. G. Skirbekk. Bergen: Universitetsforlaget, 89-93.

—— 2004. Interview with David Nash and Susan Daniel-McElroy. *Making and Placing: Abstract Sculpture, 1978–2004.* St. Ives: Tate St. Ives.

Nash, D. n.d. In *Wood Primer: the Sculpture of David Nash*, ed. L. Van Den Abeele. Essen: Galerie S65.

Strathern, M. 1991. *Partial Connections.* Maryland: Rowman & Littlefield Publishers, Inc.

Toren, C. 1995. 'Seeing the Ancestral Sites: Transformations in Fijian Notions of the Land', in *The Anthropology of Landscape: Perspectives on Place and Space,* eds. E. Hirsch and M. O' Hanlon. Oxford: Clarendon Press, 164–83.

Turnbull, D. 1996. 'Constructing Knowledge Spaces and Locating Sites of Resistance in the Modern Cartographic Transformation', in *Social Cartography: Mapping Ways of Seeing Social and Educational Change,* ed. R.G. Paulston. New York: Garland Publishing, 53–79.

—— 1998. 'Travelling Knowledge: Narratives, Assemblage and Encounters'. Unpublished manuscript, Max Planck Institute for the History of Science, Berlin.

Weiner, J.F. 2001. *Tree Leaf Talk: a Heideggerian Anthropology.* Oxford. and New York: Berg.

Chapter 6

Maps and Plans in 'Learning to See': the London Underground and Chartres Cathedral as Examples of Performing Design

David Turnbull

Introduction

Chartres Cathedral and the London Underground map are iconic examples of good design and hence are 'good to think with' – to critically interrogate our ways of seeing with. They both exemplify the way maps and plans have become the key components of the scopic regime of modernity (Jay 1988). We have learned to see the world through the drawing of lines and bounding of objects (Pickles 2004). We have learned to control and manipulate the world through its representation in the form of two-dimensional, superimposable, mobile inscriptions (Latour 1986). Maps and plans have become 'tools without which we cannot read and without which we cannot see' (Tomasch cited in Pickles 2004: 92).

In this way, according to many critics like Jay, we have become dominated by the visual. The power of this understanding of the primacy of the visual is revealed and reinforced in the representationalism of such analyses. The very mode of analysis that critiques the dominance of the visual is itself an exemplification of that dominance. An alternative analytic position is performativity which foregrounds activity and practice, and which locates seeing not just in forms and technologies of visualisation and representation, but in embodied performances and practices, situated and distributed in time and place (Hutchins 1996; Pickering 1995; Suchman 1987; Turnbull 2002).

With performativity comes the recognition of multiplicity; there are many scopic regimes in many modernities. Mapping and planning are unstable acts of bricolage: the homogenisation of messy motleys that have to be continuously renewed and stabilised (Turnbull 2003). Ways of seeing have a history and are constantly being made and institutionalised in elaborately articulated sociotechnical networks (Schivelbusch 1977). An individual's way of seeing evolves within a dynamic tradition and is shaped by the dominant technologies of vision and representation, but such ways of seeing are also social practices inseparable from the complex adaptive assemblage that is the joint interaction, engagement and movement of varieties of agents and bodies in action, in being and in knowing. An examination of the London Underground map and Chartres Cathedral provides some examples of the ways the representational and the performative speak to – and challenge – each other, especially in the tension between unity and multiplicity, homogeneity and messiness.

Both the map and the cathedral are held up as classic exemplars of unified, homogeneous style and design. Adrian Forty in his *Objects of Desire*, for example, has explicitly drawn the analogy between them in his discussion of corporate identity as a function of design (Forty 1986). Yet, on close examination of their history and construction, Chartres and the London Underground emerge as extremely heterogeneous – each of them is a motley, an ad hoc mess.

The Underground map is a piece of representational technology conceived explicitly in an advertising context to create the impression of homogeneity, whereas, though Chartres was crucially dependent on the employment of representational technology for its construction, its homogeneity is in large part a function of retrospective stylistic analysis and a modernist predilection to conceive buildings as unified, planned wholes.

The London Underground Map

If you go to the web site for the London Underground you can access a cleverly morphing, short visualisation of the London Underground map, in which the ways the map has changed shape over time are displayed and then set against supposed topographical reality. In the text the Transport Authority poses the questions: 'Has design's gain been geography's loss?' Has the map distorted our view of London?' Though it is possible to be dismissive of London Transport's self-conscious and self-serving celebration of the map as merely a marketing device, it is important to recognise the key transpositions and reversals underlying their questions and also to recognise that the map itself has brought about this self-reflection about the ways in which we have been trained to see.

When the engineering draughtsman Henry Beck first proposed the Underground map the London Passenger Transport Board was resistant, concerned that the passengers would be confused by the mismatch between the idealisations and conventions of the diagram and the geographical reality. To explore the ways in which the London Underground map has established a scopic regime, I want to revisit the history of the map's development.

The world's first underground railway line was laid in London, in 1836, running from Paddington to Farringdon. By 1906 there was a myriad of separately owned lines. All of them experienced financial difficulties and they attempted to save themselves by a scheme of through-booking to any station; by 1908 they agreed to advertise the separate lines as a single system though remaining independent. This led to the formation in 1913 of one company, the Underground Electric Railway Co. of London (UERL), which also bought most of the rival bus companies. By 1933 the government had created a monopoly – the London Passenger Transport Board (LPTB), which was dominated by UERL but in reality was an amalgamation of 165 companies (Barker and Robins 1974).

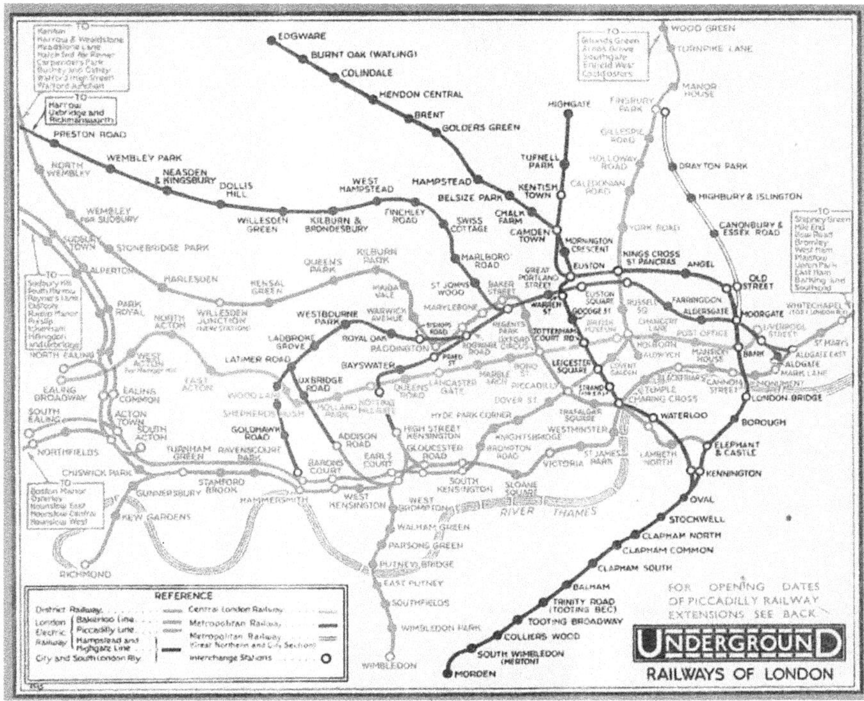

Figure 6.1 *The London Underground Map: Beck's last version 1959. Source: Figure 38, p. 48, Garland 1994.* (London Transport Museum © Transport for London)

Frank Pick, head of UERL, sometimes called the 'Lorenzo of the underground' (Forty 1979), set out to impose homogeneity on this motley mess of lines. He wanted to give the public the impression that the 'Underground railways were no longer a disparate and unplanned agglomeration of lines but that they had become part of an orderly and centrally planned system' (Forty 1986: 234). He hoped thereby to encourage more travel and to establish an integrated organisation and workforce. To this end he initiated a uniform corporate design policy, which covered every aspect of the transport system, stations, trains, personnel, architecture, signage and advertising. The aim was to show this homogeneous system as the essence of modernity and scientific management and London as a readily accessible, seamlessly connected, cornucopia of cultural, shopping and employment opportunities. A central component in Peck's campaign to train people to see the Underground as a seamless coherent network and London as an intelligible and accessible whole was the Underground Map (Figure 6.1).

This deceptively simple map, first published sixty-five years ago in 1931, has had a profound impact on the way London is seen and on the way we see in modern life. 'Of all the means by which the UERL combine changed people's ideas about the capital, none was more lasting and influential than the underground map' (Forty 1986: 237). To this day it structures the locals' and the visitors' mental map of London (see Vertesi forthcoming). Indeed it is

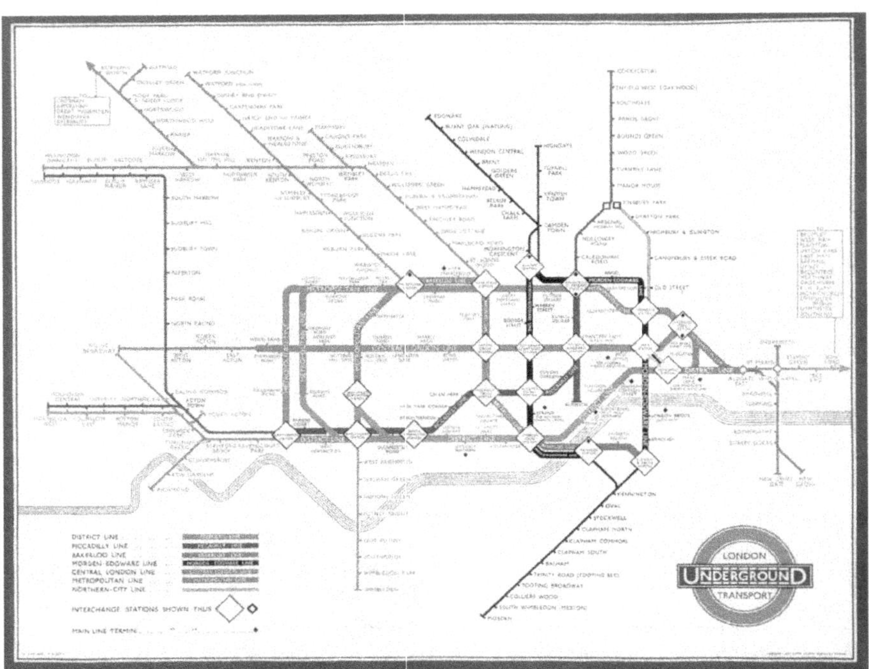

Figure 6.2 *Stingemore's last map 1932. Source: Figure 7, p. 13, Garland 1994.* (London Transport Museum © Transport for London)

now an icon of London on postcards and T-shirts. But it also established a paradigm in graphic design, which still has universal impact.

So how is this triumph of homogeneity achieved? Above all it represents the imposition of simplicity on complexity. The series of topographical maps that preceded it, culminating in F.H. Stingemore's final map, became increasingly unwieldy as the system grew and complexity increased (Figure 6.2).

In 1933, Henry Beck, in a period of unemployment, conceived the idea of substituting a schematic diagram for a map, using a 90° and 45° layout with the Central Line as a horizontal axis and with central London defined by the Circle Line:

> Looking at the old map of the Underground Railways, it occurred to me that it might be possible to tidy it up by straightening the lines, experimenting with diagonals and evening out the distance between stations. The more I thought about it the more convinced I became that the idea was worth trying, so selecting the Central London Railway as my horizontal base line, I made a rough sketch. I tried to imagine that I was using a convex lens or mirror so as to present the central area on a larger scale.
>
> The design was duly submitted, but, to my surprise and disappointment the very idea of a 45 and 90 degree schematic treatment was thought to be too 'revolutionary', my Underground map was handed back to me and that it seemed was to be the end of it. (Beck cited in Garland 1994: 17)

Though Beck's first submission was rejected out of hand by the Board in 1933, he tried again a year later and it was accepted. This dynamic interaction with the Board, which was to continue throughout Beck's career, could be caricatured as: determined genius struggles with uncomprehending bureaucratic octopus, eventually to be sidelined and die in obscurity. Beck signed away royalties and copyright in the map in 1946 in return for what he thought was lifetime design control of the map's development. This was not the Board's view; they clearly felt on occasion that they were dealing with a pedantic obsessive, and in 1960 ceased to pay any attention to Beck's attempts to have a say in the design. It is also fair to say that many of the 'improvements' that the Board imposed on Beck's map were less than felicitous (Figure 6.3).

However, this interaction with the Board was part of the dynamic through which the map developed. While Beck was always willing to incorporate new stations and lines, a constant source of contention was the display of station names and connecting stations. The last of the dramatic encounters between Beck and the Board occurred in 1960 after the Board had employed another designer, Harold Hutchinson, to update Beck's map. In the course of the exchange between Beck and the Board, while he struggled to retain control, the Board reflected their unself-conscious adoption of his design regime when they referred to 'the traditional practice associated with London Transport design of adopting broadly the 45 degree and 90 degree convention' (Garland 1994: 58) – a tradition, which of course Beck had

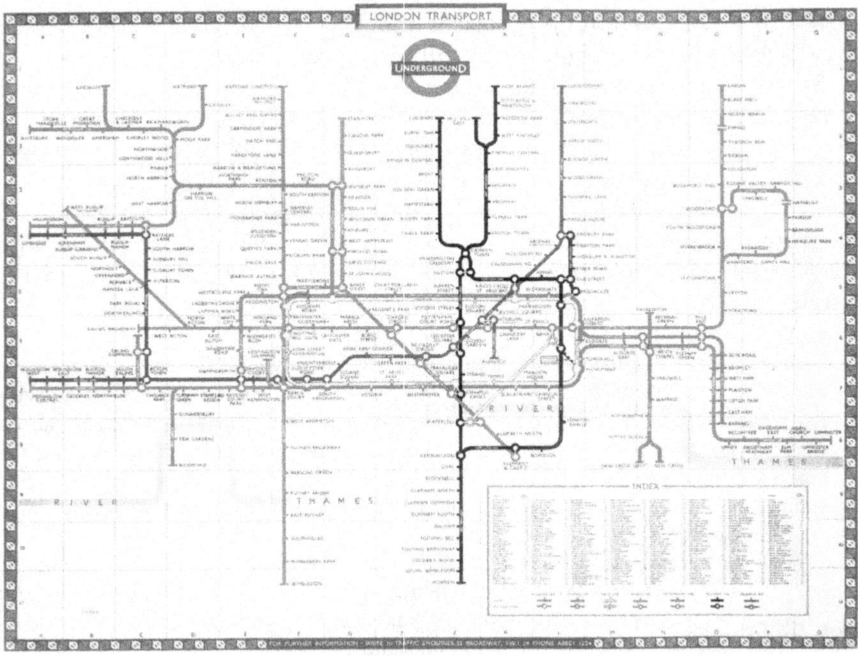

Figure 6.3 *London Transport Board's 'improvements' 1935. Source: Figure 20, p. 28, Garland 1994.* (London Transport Museum © Transport for London)

'invented' (but isn't that what traditions are, something so self-evident that they have no progenitors?) Now, of course, London Transport has become self-conscious in the postmodern way and has a museum in which Beck is celebrated as the originator of the Underground map.

Both Pick and Beck can be claimed as originator of graphic and industrial design. Pick was a founder member of the Design and Industries Association and the first chairman of the Council for Art and Design, forerunner of the present Design Council (Green 1990: 8). Beck left LPTB in 1947 and started teaching at what was to become the London School of Printing and the Graphic Arts. The notion of graphic design came in at this time, along with information and industrial design. An entire regime for focusing attention and integrating the visual into meaningful action was established, a regime based on the paradigm of Edward Johnston's 'Underground Railways Sans' typeface, which Pick introduced and which is still used throughout the system today and on Beck's Underground map (Garland 1994: 42).

The Underground map accomplishes a double homogenisation; one of the underground railway system and the other of London. By shortening outlying distances of stations and evening out inner distances it makes all journeys seem feasible. By simplifying junctions it conceals the underground reality that changing, for example, from the Northern to Circle lines at King's Cross involves two elevators, hundreds of yards of corridors and staircases, and the surface reality that St Pancras and King's Cross stations are next door to one another and the easiest thing to do is cross the street.

However, the unification of the motley of dozens of railway lines is not just a good example of representational design, it is also performative. The embodied practice of experiencing London is also transformed. The disorderly, disjointed, conglomeration of urban villages cobbled together that is the historical reality of London is homogenised into a seamless metropolis through the mediation of the map.

However, perhaps the most significant performative effect of the diagram, in the context of trying to understand the practices that constitute the Underground, is the way it structures 'a shared interactional space' of the kind Lucy Suchman (Suchman 1987) talks about and which Kathryn Henderson discusses in her accounts of the way engineers use drawings. Henderson argues that drawings allow for 'collective cognition' because they permit 'multiple interpretations within a common schema as opposed to a unified rational process determined by a fixed representation' (Henderson 1991: 457). Roth, in his similar work on the collective construction of the interpretation of graphs, argues: 'Perception is instantiated not primarily in the brain, but rather in the social practices enacted over and about the unfolding graphical displays' (Roth 2003: 19).

This is also apparent in the work of Christian Heath and Paul Luff on the 'invisible work' of the infrastructure in the control rooms of the Underground. They show that the management of the moment-to-moment running of the system depends on the interactions of a Line Controller, who manages the running of the trains and is guardian of the timetable, and a Divisional Information Assistant (DIA), who communicates with passengers and station managers. The two coordinate the running of the Bakerloo Line using computers, telephones etc., but most especially through 'seeing' a line diagram, which shows the movements of the trains in real time, and the paper timetable, which integrates all the details and variations to do with things like crews, maintenance, bomb scares and announcements of train times. The Controller and the DIA have to coordinate their activities in running the trains in a situation where they are constantly changing components of the system, but don't have time to tell each other what they are doing. Instead they develop a system of seeing and hearing each other in action. Each overhears the other's phone conversations and 'sees' the other 'seeing' the line diagram. They perform their own jobs and simultaneously monitor the other's (Heath and Luff 1992). It's a form of performativity and distributed vision; the seeing of seeing in a space structured around modes of representation.

Chartres Cathedral

Suchman has pointed out: 'the view, that purposeful action is determined by plans, is deeply rooted in the Western human sciences as *the* correct model of the rational actor' (Suchman 1987: ix). Similarly drawings are held to be the *sine qua non* of design as maps are for navigation. Nowhere is this representationalist presupposition more evident than in the question of how the great Gothic cathedrals like Chartres were designed and built. The question is contentious and problematic; in the first instance, because, in the case of Chartres, there are no plans and no known architect. There has been a tendency on the part of historians to make it a mystery and to create a great

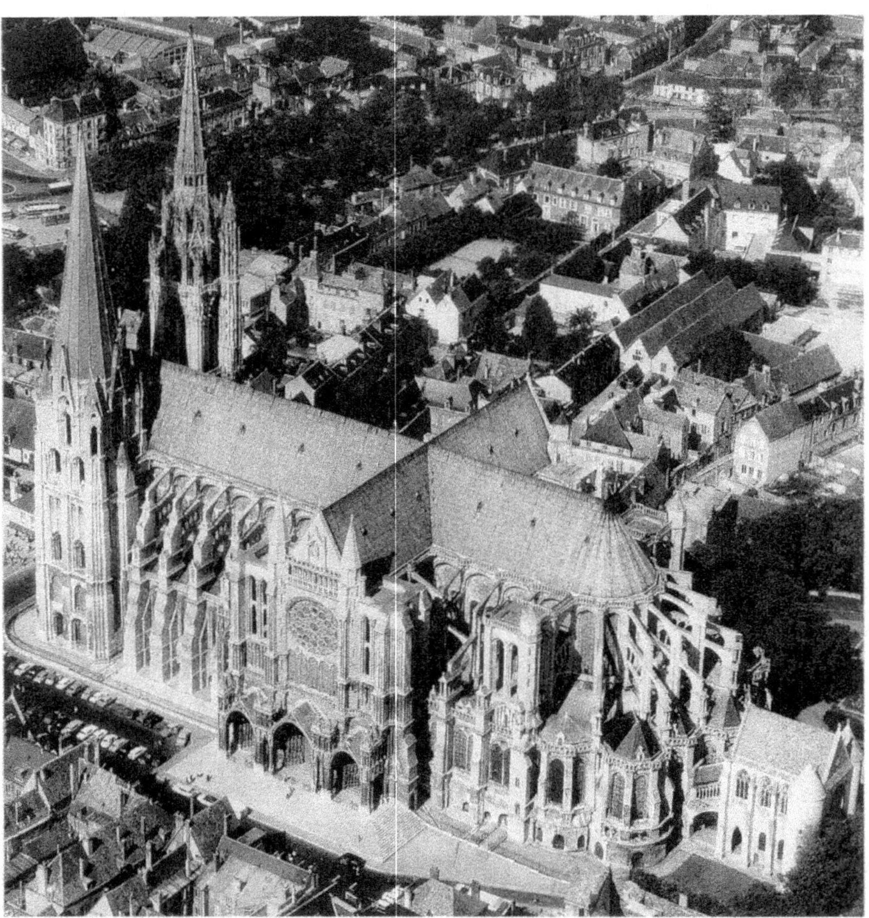

Figure 6.4 *Chartre's messiness and incompleteness: the two west towers are completely different, and sites for a further seven towers have never been filled.* (Photo: D. Turnbull)

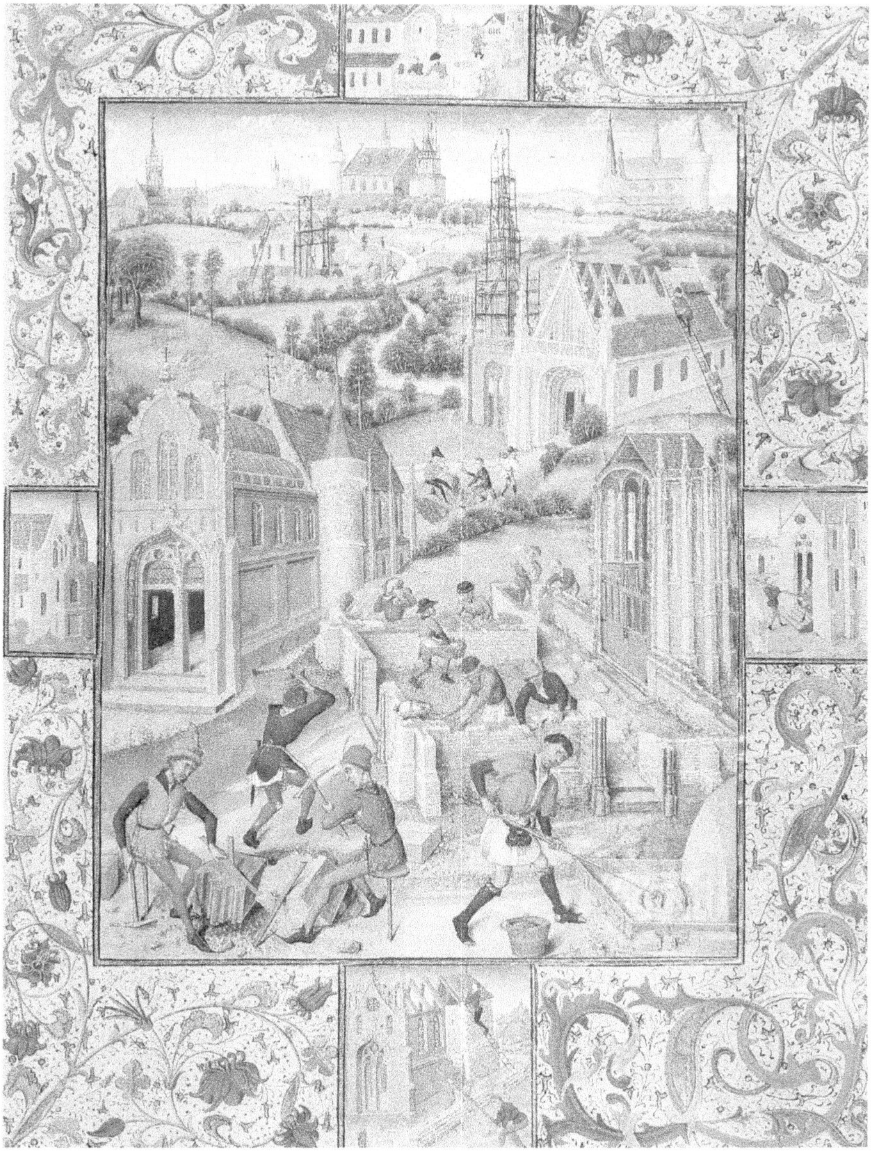

Figure 6.5 *Cathedrals result from the work of many men. Source: Figure 49, p. 48, Coldstream 1991.* (Osterreichische Nationalbibliotek Wien)

divide between then and now, by either attributing secret knowledge to the masons or special building skills now lost. Alternatively, historians have denied any divide and any historicity by asserting that they must have had plans. Such explanatory strategies now stand in need of revision thanks to the detailed analysis of the structure of Chartres by the Australian architectural historian John James. Chartres has been held up as a glorious example of Gothic architecture, a harmonious unity embodying light, spirituality, innovation and complexity. For James, Chartres remains the epitome of twelfth-century architectural spirituality; with soaring height and sumptuous glass walls, it still has the innovative flying buttresses and the complexity of pinnacles and spires, but where there was unity and coherence he reveals 'an ad hoc mess' (James 1982: 9) (Figure 6.4).

As is obvious, once you break with the notion of a 'Gothic style' guiding the design, Chartres has a bewildering variety of spires, pinnacles, buttresses, fliers, roofs, doors and windows. Rather less obvious, but more important in structural terms, the bays and the axes in the nave and transepts are completely irregular, the only regularity being in the interior elevation. James's brick-by-brick, moulding-by-moulding analysis shows there to have been thirteen major design and structural changes in the unusually rapid

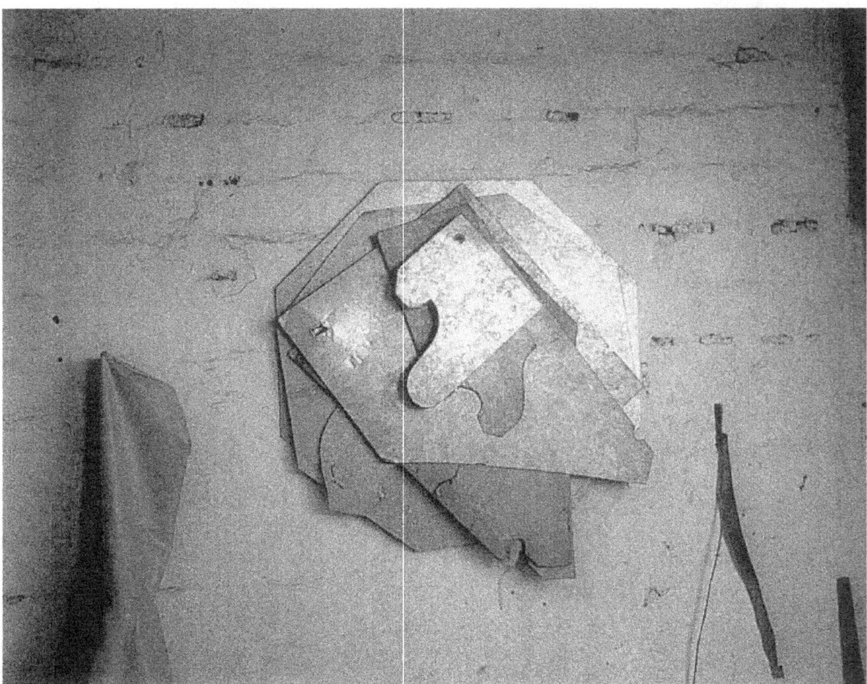

Figure 6.6 *Modern templates exactly like medieval ones in use by stonemasons at Melbourne University.* (Photo: D. Turnbull)

process of rebuilding between 1194 and 1230, undertaken following a disastrous fire. James finds that there were nine different contractors or master masons, and that there was no overall designer, just a succession of builders. 'Chartres was the *ad hoc* accumulation of the work of many men' (James 1982: 123) (Figure 6.5). James's claim that there was no one architect has been contested but the argument lies beyond the scope of this chapter. However, his identification of major design changes are very telling, as are the other factors which he points out: the lack of plans, the lack of a common measure and the crucial role of templates (Figures 6.6 and 6.7).

The question of the apparent lack of plans is extremely important and contentious (see Turnbull 2003). While there were site drawings – that is, full-scale outlines on the floor of specific parts of the building – no plans, in the modern sense of scaled blue prints of the whole, were used to build Chartres Cathedral. However, such is the dominance of the plan/map-based scopic regime, that the representationalist mindset of many historians leads them to claim that buildings of such innovation and complexity *must* have had plans. What a performative approach suggests is that plans and maps are devices for moving, assembling, transmitting and storing knowledge that are embedded in a range of supporting practices. Rather than preceding and determining cathedral building, maps and plans were developed in response to changes in the socioeconomic system and its accompanying knowledge spaces; in the case of the cathedrals, in the course of the building process itself. The cathedrals and their building systems co-evolved in a complex adaptive system (Lansing 2003).

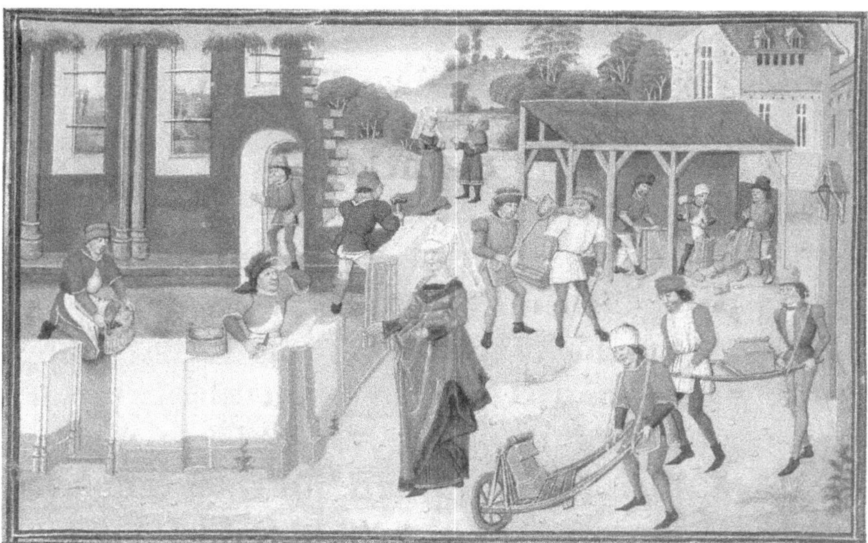

Figure 6.7 *A Masons' lodge. Source: Figure 8, p. 10, Coldstream 1991.* Bibliotheque Royale de Belgique Albert 1e Brussels (ms 6 fol 554 v).

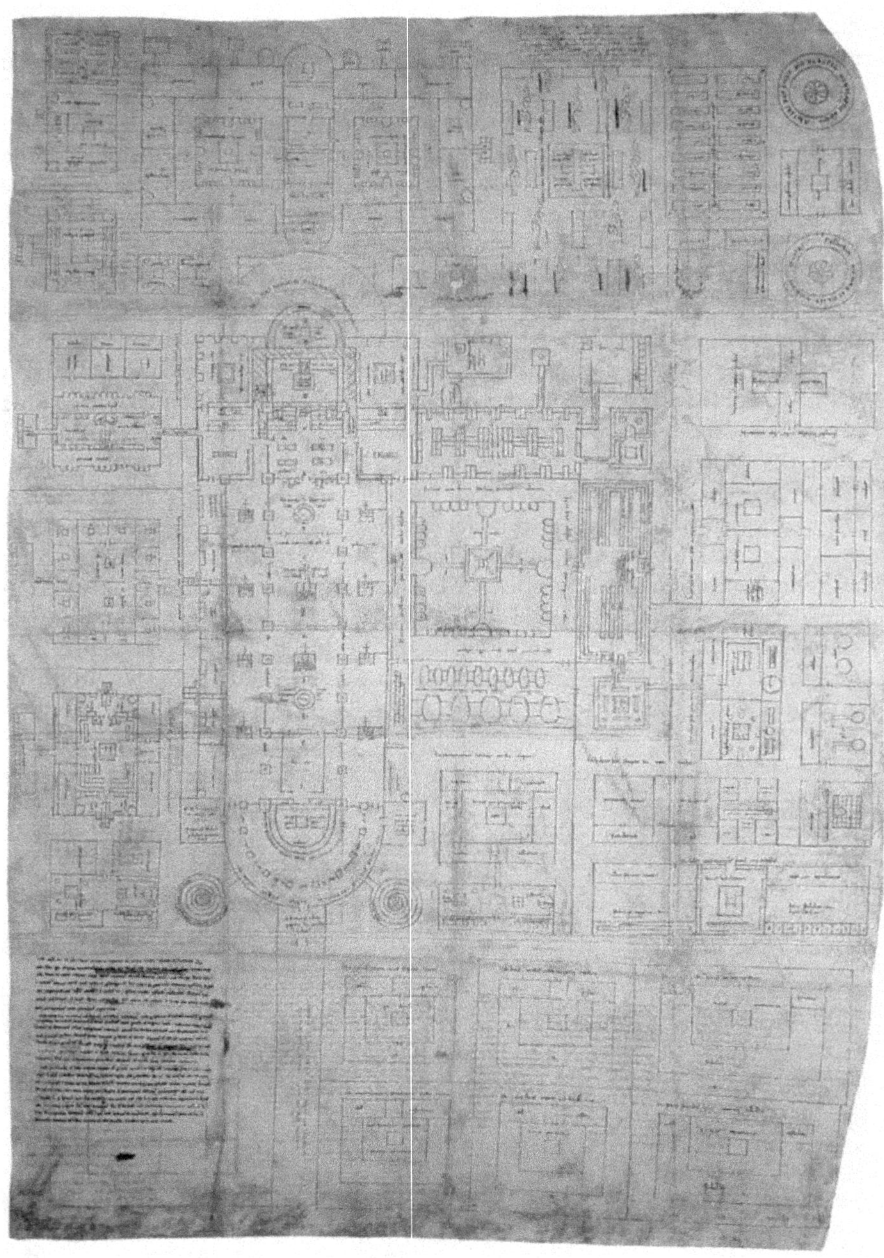

Figure 6.8 *The plan of St Gall 820 AD. Source: Figure 9, p. 14, Harvey, 1991.* (London: The British Library, 1991. Stiftsbibliothek St. Gallen)

The medieval historian Mary Carruthers' painstaking analysis of medieval knowledge production reveals that for the scholastics memory has a spatiotemporal structure dependent on location and ordering in the past. In the pursuit of understanding and remembering the liturgy, the early medieval scholars developed rhetoric as a creative art for meditation and thinking. It was a craft knowledge for storing memories and thought and inventing new insight and understanding. It was a skilled visual practice based in location (Carruthers 1998: 10ff.).

In the scopic regime of the medieval world, the earliest extant plan is that of St Gall AD 820 (Figure 6.8) but on Carruthers' account it was not a blueprint for an intended construction, it was a 'meditational instrument', and furthermore cathedrals were not just masterpieces of religious architecture but 'machines for thinking' (Carruthers 1998: 228, 276). What counts as seeing, knowing and remembering changes as the construction process evolves, as is evidenced by the transformation of the mason from master builder to architect. The first indication of the notion that plans are like sets of instructions to be traced or copied comes with the earliest mention of a tracing house attached to a cathedral construction in 1274, which is the zenith, not the beginning, of the cathedral crusade (Branner 1963: 131).

Cathedral building precipitated an economic transformation so extensive that clerics adopted different technologies and 'sites of memory'; rather than use them as meditational devices for memorising the liturgy, they collected site documents in the vestry and used plans for discussing future projects (Erlande-Brandenburg 1994: 257). The previous memory regime and practices were supplanted; plans and maps became the key control devices, synonymous with seeing and knowing.

If, as the balance of evidence would seem to suggest, architectural drawings to control the design process were developed during the great cathedral building period, how is it possible that a large proportion of the Gothic cathedrals were built without them? The achievement of the order of complexity and structural innovation involved in the construction of the cathedrals required a high degree of precision in the production of the stones and it also required larger numbers of workers as well as a greater variety of types of workers to act in coordination. These factors created production and organisational difficulties that turn crucially on a fundamental problem – communication. Knowledge and instructions had to move between many participants. For a given building there had to be clear communication between the ecclesiastical client and the master mason, and between the master and other masons on and off site, since some stones are cut at the quarry. Masons had also to communicate with other teams of masons and other workers, principally carpenters, who were responsible for the invisible but nonetheless essential scaffolding and form work, as well as the roof and all the heavy lifting equipment. In addition, knowledge had to be transmitted between sites and across successive generations of masons. The key communication device is the template, a pattern or mould that permits both the accurate cutting and replication of shaped stone and the transmission of know1edge between workers (Harvey 1972: 119, 174). The power of the template lies not only in the way in which it facilitates accurate mass production, but also in the fact that simple geometrical rules of thumb will often suffice for the template itself to be accurately reproduced as often as required (James 1982: 34; James 1979 vol. 11: 543). The template helps to make possible the unified organisation of large numbers of men with varied training and skill over considerable periods of time.

On them were encapsulated every design decision that had to be passed down to the men doing the carving in shop and quarry. Through them the work of all the masons on the site was controlled and coordinated. With them dozens, and in some cases hundreds, of men were guided to a common purpose. They were the primary instruments of the trade (James 1989: 2; Shelby 1971).

Though templates were essential representational devices, other more performative elements were also essential; talk, tradition, and trial and error. Masonry as a tradition, contrary to popular myth and the desires of Freemasons, did not have any secret knowledge. But, the tradition did differ in two important ways from that of other organised trades whose skills and practices were handed on through guilds and apprenticeships, both of which made masonry literally an 'ad hoc' profession. Firstly, they seldom practised their profession in one place: the job did not come to them, they went to the job (Shelby 1976). This exposure to new sites and the work of others was a

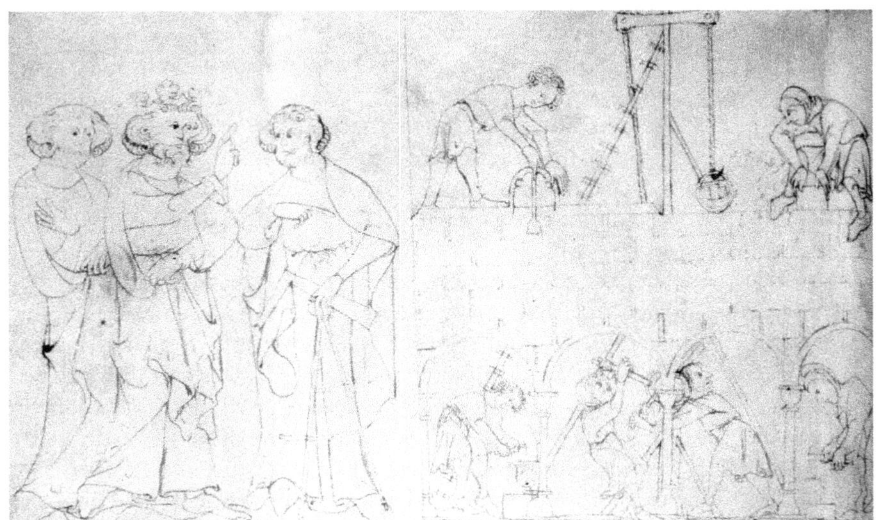

Figure 6.9 *The master mason and the clients talking. Source: Figure 10, p. 12, Coldstream 1991. (*By Permission of The British Library Cotton Nero D1 f. 23v)

constant spur to innovation. Secondly, the construction site was essentially an experimental laboratory in which they were able to try and see whether an innovation was successful. For example, close observation of the drying mortar enabled the builders to detect areas of stress in the fabric and to take appropriate remedial measures through the placement of buttresses, pinnacles or reinforcement (Mark 1982: 56).

This, then, leaves the question of who designed Chartres and the other medieval churches, given that there were no architects in the modern sense (their role developing along with the development of plans and the gradual separation of theory from practice). Or, to put it another way, in the absence of plans how did the church and the craft traditions work together? The patron bishop couldn't build, and the master mason couldn't read, so how did the spiritual and intellectual values of the day become incorporated in the structure (Shelby 1970)? Lon Shelby's deceptively simple, but profoundly important, answer is 'talk' (Figure 6.9).

Frequent – sometimes daily – consultations between the master mason and the patron or his representative were the normal routine in medieval building. It was 'this symbiotic relationship' which provides an essential clue to who designed the medieval churches (Shelby 1970: 18, fn 48). It was this dynamic interaction that enabled radical innovations as well as the constant design changes, but it was the use of constructive geometry in the drawing of the templates that allowed the masons to make their own templates incorporating their own specific design elements (Shelby 1981). Talk, tradition and templates provided for a distributed and situated design process. The design as well as the construction of the cathedral was indeed the resulted of 'the ad hoc accumulation of the work of many men'.

Conclusion

From a performative perspective, the map and the cathedral are examples of distributed design where the achievement of homogeneity in a welter of heterogeneity serves to create new knowledge spaces in which people, skills and technical devices interact, co-producing cognitive and social order. From a representationalist perspective the cathedral and the map exemplify the centrality of the concept of a plan and design style in shaping the way we see. Each of these perspectives is self-exemplifying and neither is more valid or fundamental than the other. Since we cannot avoid seeing the world through the ways we construct it and analyse it, holding the contrasting perspectives in dynamic tension with each other is both an effective way of reflexively including our own performance and representation of intelligibility and visuality, and a more powerful heuristic for understanding the ways we see, shape and order the world.

References

Barker, T.C. and M. Robins, 1974. *A History of London Transport: Passenger Travel and the Development of the Metropolis*. Vol. 11: *The Twentieth Century to 1970.* London: George Allen and Unwin.

Branner, R. 1963. 'Villard de Honnecourt, Reims and the Origin of Gothic Architectural Drawing', *Gazette des Beaux-Arts* 61: 129–46.

Carruthers, M. 1998. *The Craft of Thought: Meditation, Rhetoric and the Making of Images, 400–1200*. Cambridge: Cambridge University Press.

Coldstream, N. 1991. *Masons and Sculptors*. London: British Museum Press.

Erlande-Brandenburg, A. 1994. *The Cathedral: The Social and Architectural Dynamics of Construction*. Cambridge: Cambridge University Press.

Forty, A. 1979. 'Lorenzo of the Underground', *London Journal* 5 (1): 113–19.

—— 1986. *Objects of Desire: Design and Society, 1875–1980*. London: Thames and Hudson.

Garland, K. 1994. *Mr Beck's Underground Map*. Harrow Weald: Capital Transport.

Grasseni, C. 2004 'Skilled Vision. An Apprenticeship in Breeding Aesthetics', *Social Anthropology* 12 (1): 1–15.

Green, O. 1990. *Underground Art: London Transport Posters, 1908 to the Present*. London: Studio Vista.

Harvey, J. 1972. *The Medieval Architect*. London: Wayland Press.

—— 1974. *Cathedrals of England and Wales*. London: B.T. Batsford.

Harvey, P.D.A. 1991 *Medieval Maps*. London: British Library

Heath, C. and P. Luff. 1992. 'Collaboration and Control: Crisis Management and Multimedia Technology in London Underground Control Rooms', *Computer Supported Cooperative Work (CSCW)* 1: 69–94.

Henderson, Kathryn. 1991. 'Flexible Sketches and Inflexible Databases: Visual Communication, Conscription Devices, and Boundary Objects in Design Engineering', *Science, Technology and Human Values* 16: 448–73.

Hutchins, E. 1996. *Cognition in the Wild*. Cambridge, Mass.: MIT Press.

James, J. 1979. *The Contractors of Chartres*, 2 vols. Wyong: Mandorla Publications.

—— 1982. *Chartres: The Masons Who Built a Legend*. London: Routledge and Kegan Paul.

—— 1989. *The Template-Makers of the Paris Basin*. Leura: West Grinstead Nominees.

Jay, M. 1988. 'Scopic Regimes of Modernity', in *Vision and Visuality*. H. Foster. Seattle: Bay Press: 3–23.

Lansing, J.S. 2003. 'Complex Adaptive Systems', *Annual Review of Anthropology* 32: 183–204.

Latour, Bruno. 1986. 'Visualisation and Cognition: Thinking With Eyes and Hands', *Knowledge and Society* 6: 1–40.

Mark, R. 1982. *Experiments in Gothic Structure*. Cambridge, Mass.: MIT Press.

Pickering, A. 1995. *The Mangle of Practice: Time, Agency, and Science*. Chicago: University of Chicago Press.

Pickles, J. 2004. *A History of Spaces: Cartographic Reason, Mapping and the Geo-coded World*. London: Routledge.

Roth, W.-M. 2003. *Towards an Anthropology of Graphing: Semiotic and Activity Theory Perspectives*. Dordrecht: Kluwer Academic Publishers.

Schivelbusch, W. 1977. *The Railway Journey: the Industrialisation of Time and Space*. Leamington Spa: Berg.
Shelby, L.R. 1970. 'The Education of Medieval English Master Masons', *Medieval Studies* 32: 1–26.
—— 1971. 'Medieval Masons' Templets', *Journal of the Society of Architectural Historians* XXX: 140–52.
—— 1976. 'The "Secret" of the Medieval Masons', in *On Pre-Modern Technology and Science*, eds. B. Hall and D. West. Malibu: Undena Publications, 201–22.
—— 1981. 'The Contractors of Chartres, [review], *GESTA* XX: 173–78.
Suchman, L. 1987. *Plans and Situated Actions: The Problem of Human-Machine Communication*. Cambridge: Cambridge University Press.
Turnbull, D. 2002. 'Performance and Narrative, Bodies and Movement in the Construction of Places and Objects, Spaces and Knowledges: The Case of The Maltese Megaliths', *Theory, Culture and Society* 19 (5&6): 125–43.
—— 2003. *Masons, Tricksters and Cartographers: Comparative Studies in the Sociology of Scientific and Indigenous Knowledge*, 2nd edn. London: Routledge.
Vertesi, J. forthcoming. 'Mind the Gap. The London Underground Map and Users' Representations of Urban Space', *Social Studies of Science*.

Part III

The Social Schooling of the Eye in Scientific and Medical Settings

Chapter 7

CT Suite: Visual Apprenticeship in the Age of the Mechanical Viewbox

Barry Saunders

'CT suite' is the conventional term for the cluster of rooms, in English-speaking hospitals of any size, that houses a computed tomography scanner and its controls, a waiting area, a reading station.[1] But the term 'suite' is of interest for more archaic connotations: persons and practices *following* one another (*suivant*) in and among these rooms. The earliest suites were courtly entourages. What passes today through the rooms of the CT suite is still a drama of prestige and hierarchy, division of labour, mannered performance.

Apprenticeship is of course more than ceremonial following. It is a political and economic arrangement in which labour is exchanged for training in a craft. Some parts of apprenticeship involve following: emulation, copying, in the master's workshop.

However, following need not be slavish imitation. The CT suite's masters are engaged in a kind of following themselves: diagnosis has long been associated with tracking and hunting, and with divination (Ginzburg 1989). Such practices draw on cunning and interpretive acumen. In the CT suite, radiologists are hunters and priests, pursuing malign agencies of disease, reading shadows of entrails.

So the trainees whose apprenticeship experiences are the focus of this chapter – radiology 'residents' in a US university hospital – are thus doubly in pursuit: they follow expertise in following. They are apprentices in the priestly craft of reading in pursuit of culprit lesions. There are other lesser apprentices too. To the extent that some of these residents' learning experiences are shared on occasion by clinicians and others among radiology's clients, 'apprenticeship' as a form of radiological learning is distributed beyond the radiological guild.[2] Indeed, my own positions as ethnographic participant observer were informed at many levels by structures of apprenticeship.[3]

Not all radiological learning is adequately summarised by the rubric of 'apprenticeship'. To be sure, hierarchies of hospital-based physician learning and service – from supervising attending, to fellow, to resident, to student – are roughly analogous to systems of indentured or paid servitude in craft guilds: residents and students work as apprentices, fellows as journeymen, soon to seek qualification as masters in their own right. But in residency programmes, multiple trainees owe allegiance to many masters simultaneously, and not all choose a particular mentor.[4] Nor do all structures of knowledge transmission presume, or follow the contours of, master–trainee relations.

Pursuit in the CT suite: this should not be understood as a kind of lyricism. Radiological diagnosis has a substantial tolerance for – indeed, capitalises upon – discontinuity. Radiological interpretation in teaching hospitals is remarkably disjoint, interrupted. This is partly due to the structure of the 'docket', i.e., seriation of cases. It is partly due to rhythms of 'rotation' in radiological labour and training, along multiple professional axes: radiology, nursing, radiation technology, administration, technical support. And it is due to other competing hospital agendas. Historically, the CT scanner itself has contributed to shopfloor discontinuity – in part through stimulus of subspecialisation.[5] Interruption has important implications for radiological pedagogy. Relations of teachers and learners are sometimes intensified but frequently challenged and foreshortened by the staccato and irregular rhythm of workday tasks in CT.

Learning to read CT scans is part of the process of learning to read medical images in general.[6] A substantial part of radiological teaching is didactic – authoritative presentations delivered to groups in lecture-hall settings. And another portion of radiological learning is autodidactic, i.e., rote memorisation of information codified in textbooks, atlases and protocols. But there is a major component of radiological pedagogy that is interactive, teacher-on-learner, involving both exemplary demonstrations and situated critique of novice performance – important aspects of apprenticeship.

In the reading room, one of the two fourth-year medical students on service is now the keeper of the logbook, dutifully inscribing findings as the team clusters around the fellow, reviewing studies together. Suddenly the films on 'the board' lurch to the right, and keep moving – until the student realises he has accidentally pushed the corner of the logbook into the motor switch.

Student 1: Oh, dear.
Student 2: [*Laughing*]
CT Fellow: [*Laughing*] When I was a resident, that used to happen all the time and I used to feel like such a dork all the time for doing that.

Students: [*Laughing*]
Fellow: Hoo hoo, huh, there goes the board, now everybody's lookin' at ya like, what are you doing? And [*laughing*] you're like, I don't have a clue. [*Laughing*] And the board's just goin' by. [*Laughing*] And you're just sittin' there with that stupid look on your face.
Student 1: Dowee.
Student 2: You're in charge of the book …
Fellow: And your chairman's lookin' at ya like he can't believe he accepted you into the program … [*laughing*] You get used to it after awhile.

The cluelessness of trainees, practice under criticism, learning from observed mistakes, begrudging acceptance by the master: ingredients of apprenticeship.

Social Structures of Pedagogy

Salient among the social conditions of radiological teaching are facts of rank and specialty. First, the hierarchy of roles.

- *Medical students* (most of whom do not become radiologists) spend four weeks in a radiology 'clerkship' during their clinical years of medical school. They also learn image interpretation skills while on other specialty rotations. Some of these specialties, like neurology or ENT (ear-nose-throat) surgery, are indeed rather CT-intensive. Students in radiology clerkships receive a core of dedicated group instruction, but in shopfloor settings they tend to perform support tasks – like collation of patient data.
- *Residents* spend four years in radiology residency – following one prior training year in another discipline, such as pathology or medicine – and then they become eligible to sit for the national certification exam in diagnostic radiology. Residencies are divided into month-long rotations on different services across the radiological enterprise: chest, GI (gastrointestinal), nuclear medicine, etc. CT scans are represented on several of these rotations – notably, neuroradiology (where brain CT scans are interpreted alongside MRIs (magnetic resonance images) and other head/neck studies), body CT, paediatric imaging. Throughout training, all residents go to frequent conferences: daily noon teaching conferences, biweekly 'hotseat' conferences, and any interdisciplinary conferences proper to their current assignments. The more interactive of these conferences include, for trainees, episodes of apprenticeship, performances under criticism. But the most important sites for assumption of apprenticeship roles are on the radiological shopfloor—especially in the reading rooms, elbow-to-elbow with mentors (fellow or attending), where residents practise, far more actively than medical students, the production of 'readings'.

- *Fellows,* journeyman of the radiology guild, have already completed a radiology residency (usually elsewhere). A fellowship comprises two years of further training in a particular subspecialty, and opportunity to practise with more autonomy, while still under supervision. Fellows assume considerable responsibility for teaching residents and students, and thus often function as mentors in apprenticeship relations. They learn and teach in conferences.
- *Attending* radiologists are the masters. Each contributes some particular subspecialty expertise to complement that of the full faculty. A few radiology faculty members are non-physicians, holding doctorates in physics, computer science, or other fields – thus are removed from diagnosis and its teaching. Some attendings have research/publication commitments in addition to service and teaching responsibilities; other attendings are non-academic, i.e., not held to research agendas – though they may be quite active in teaching and mentoring. Attendings all rotate through a duty roster that assigns responsibilities for supervision of particular radiological services (e.g., body CT) a day or two at a time, and thus are, in aggregate, responsible for all official image readings in the hospital. They also share responsibility for periodic conduct of teaching conferences. And they mentor residents and fellows, in interactive conference settings and at reading room viewboxes.

This radiological hierarchy continually reproduces itself, as individuals ascend within it. This occurs in explicit and codified ways – for instance, competency examinations punctuating each career. The hierarchy also takes

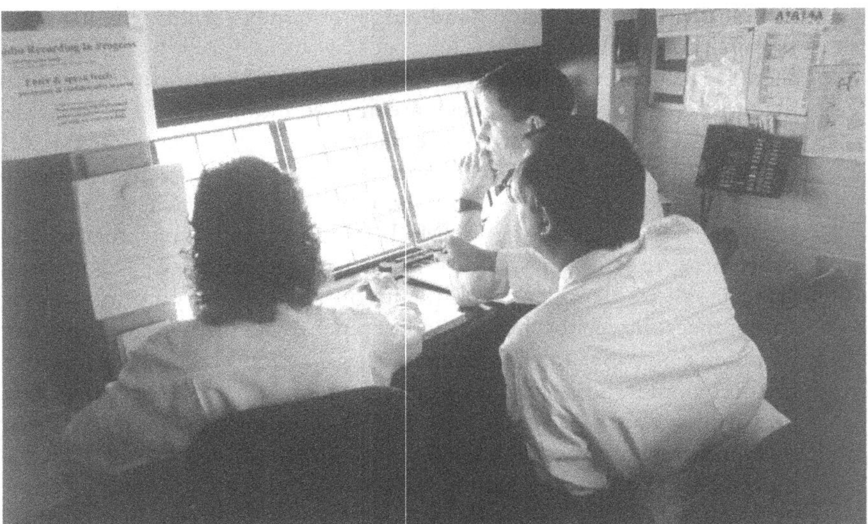

Figure 7.1 *Pedagogy at the viewbox.*

shape in tacit, implicit ways. It is often visible in seating arrangements – at teaching conferences, as well as at the reading room viewbox. One attending sits at conspicuous remove from the film, as if to dramatise his keen vision, while granting trainees a close view (Figure 7.1); other attendings insist that a resident sit between them and the phone, to insulate them from interruption.

Teaching is distributed across all levels of the radiological hierarchy. Attendings and fellows teach residents, who in turn teach students. All but the students teach client clinicians who come to the reading room. Often they learn from these client clinicians as well.

In addition to hierarchy, the crucial fact of specialisation, and thus cross-disciplinary communication, informs radiological teaching. Whether instruction unfolds in departmental contexts or between radiologists and their clinical (non-radiologist) colleagues, it is often challenged to bridge specificities of expertise.

The Body CT attending *du jour* sees, on the reading room viewbox, what she believes to be clot in a pulmonary artery – but she cannot, on the phone, convince the clinician (an oncologist), who notes that his patient is only mildly short of breath. The Body CT attending calls in a colleague expert in interpretation of thin-slice chest CT; he in turn phones back the oncologist.

> Hi, Owen, this is Hank. [*pause*] As Crista said ... he indeed has very extensive thrombus within his pulmonary artery. He basically has a saddle embolus ... You can actually follow these thrombi down to both lower pulmonary arteries. [*pause*] To me there's no question ... Crista said something about angio. I really feel very strongly that doesn't need to be done ...

In some such dialogues, the reciprocal exchange of specialty insight, in face of constructive but critical appraisals, exemplifies how vectors of apprenticeship-style teaching can point in both directions. And the agonistic features of some consultations suggest that mastery is something that cannot necessarily be presumed, but must be continually performed and re-established.

If apprenticeship requires repeated daily contact in routines of work, the best model in CT (Neuro or Body) is the relation of resident to fellow, since they both work together on the service for the duration of a month. Attendings, on the other hand, rotate on a daily basis, such that a half-dozen may work in CT over the course of a month – and in any case they are often more removed from the daily routines of film handling. If, on the other hand, what is important to apprenticeship is mimesis of exemplary performance, and practice under particularised criticism, then much viewbox work by any trainer/trainee pair is apprenticeship.

Some skills are learned quickly by residents – consistent with the commonplace maxim often voiced about learning manual procedures: 'see one, do one, teach one'. There is a bit of bravado in this, and it defies notions of apprenticeship that involve more repetition, patience, practice – but there is also plenty of slow learning in radiology, especially at the viewbox.

Radiological knowledge is accumulated incrementally, over many cases, and involves emulation of thought styles, ways of speaking – as in presentations and dictations. For instance, proper ways to express diagnostic equivocation: a lesion is 'suggestive of' something; or 'could be consistent with' something. Many of the 'pearls' of this kind of craft-knowing are not laws that are readily systematised, but are more modest rules of thumb that are context-dependent and find their way into trainees' funds of tacit knowledge.

Pedagogical Settings

Perhaps the most consistent setting for teaching and learning of radiological visual skills is the teaching conference. It takes place at the same time every day, and offers brief refuge from the press of clinical urgencies on various radiological services. On especially busy days, residents' attendance at these conferences is enabled by fellows or attendings willing to pick up their load and work through the lunch hour. Indeed, residents and students – and faculty – who attend often eat their lunches in conference.

Teaching conferences are quite flexible as learning venues. All are orchestrated around images – slides, films, Powerpoint. Some are thoroughly didactic – covering topics that the presenters are qualified to address, and unfolding according to highly rationalised structures. Other conferences are organised by cases – selected and ordered according to particular criteria, but each bearing its own lessons and logics. Conferences that unfold as case series resemble in some ways a day's work at the viewbox (Figure 7.2).

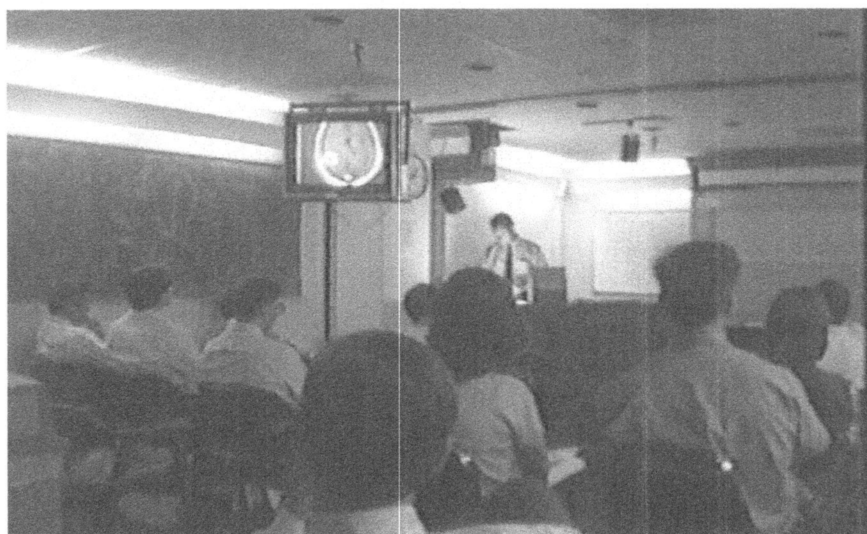

Figure 7.2 *A teaching conference.*

Often didactic presentations are delivered as parallel slide shows – using matching projectors. This is a presentation mode *de rigeur* at national and international conferences – for instance, the annual RSNA (Radiological Society of North America) conference in Chicago. A side-by-side projection format permits juxtapositions of one slice with another, one patient with another, one imaging modality with another, before with after, image with diagram, image with text. The hinge of juxtaposition – radiologists call it 'correlation' – is an eminently plastic one, and one that underwrites all radiological thought and practice.

It is the case series conferences which generate the most apprenticeship-like engagements of learners and teachers. Whoever is running a conference, the assembler and custodian of the case docket (it can be a resident, but in many conferences and in all 'hotseat' conferences, the attending presides), introduces each case and chooses someone to be the case discussant. Unlike some teaching conferences in other clinical domains, like the CPC (clinical-pathological conference) of internal medicine, where the role of discussant is an honour bestowed on a senior clinician (Eddy and Clanton 1982, Hunter 1991), in radiological teaching conferences, the discussant is often a resident. The attending's approach with a resident is often interrogative. Each step of the resident's effort – finding a lesion, describing it, considering what disease entities might take such an appearance, and then judging their relative likelihood – is subject to challenges, deflections, interruptions from the attending.

'What do you see?' asks the attending. Time for Norman, standing in front of the assembled conference goers, to summarise his findings. He begins with the plain abdominal contrast study:

> ... small bowel followthrough showing nice contrast in terminal ileum ... narrowing of terminal ileum and some filling defects ... ulceration ... Along here – a question of a fistulous tract between terminal ileum and sigmoid colon. I don't know if you can appreciate that. In addition ... linear contrast ... could be consistent with pseudopolyps ...

The attending interrupts in a peremptory voice: 'This is not pseudopolyp ... This is Crohns, with effaced narrowed small bowel ...'

Norman resumes his description – though the attending has contradicted his previous testimony, supplied a new and briefer description, and indeed has already shortcircuited to a final diagnosis.

> ... air-filled terminal ileum, you can see how that wraps down ... whoops, too dark [*the display*] ... loss of normal *valvulae conniventes*, and normal mucosal [*pauses, unable to remember proper term*], mucosal, ah [*pauses—discomfiture produces chuckles from others*], features.

The attending contradicts again: 'That's just debris in front of the stricture.'

For all the attending's brusqueness, Norman is actually doing well. He returns to 'a nice demonstration of a fistulous connection'. The attending seems pleased, and asks him to 'look at the CT'. Norman displays one CT film and adjusts magnification to show just a few slices. He slides the film to display images sequentially.

> ... start to see on this image – that there is ... transverse colon is coming across here ... bowel wall a bit thickened ... colon is not compressed yet ... more evident further down [*serial images*] ... You kind of get this inflammatory mass in the right lower quadrant ... further down ... there is stranding ... Contrast cannot get into this area because of all the inflammatory changes ... It's tracking down that whole area ... actually it's pretty neat – we can see that area of fistulous connection ... It sort of looks like a tornado ...

At this last there is a faint murmur from one side of the room, perhaps reaction to the informal tone or fanciful simile, as if it were somehow presumptuous, or inviting of further contradiction.

The resident is finished, and the last word is left to the attending. He summarises succinctly: 'a pretty classic case of Crohns, both from GI as well as CT findings'. For all the tones of refutation, he has mostly ratified the resident's account.

When Norman has returned to his seat, and while the attending is scanning the room for the next victim, a resident sitting behind Norman leans forward. 'Was that fun, Norman?'

Two important theatrical devices operate in case conferences. One is that of *inquisition* – intensified in 'hotseat' conferences, like this one – in which the resident's role resembles that of courtroom witness, and the attending plays a kind of cross-examiner. The hotseat format is calculated to challenge, to expose indecision and error in diagnostic process, to inculcate poise under pressure. Its agonistic dynamic draws upon, and harkens toward, both courtroom conventions and competitive relations with clinical colleagues.

A second prominent device is that of *intrigue*. Sometimes the instant case has intrinsically puzzling dimensions. In teaching conferences, however, often these puzzling dimensions are a function of some kind of artifice, especially withholding. The attending does not offer the clinical context; or s/he only provides limited portions of an imaging study; or s/he withholds the tissue diagnosis that is written on the case folder; or s/he offers counterfactual information: 'OK, same picture, different patient.' These concealments and supplements are tactical, calculated to summon particular diagnostic efforts from a resident addressing a case – a more expanded list of possible diagnostic entities; an explanation for incongruous findings. (More on intrigue below.)

Outside conferences most radiological teaching happens at the reading room viewboxes. This is so for students and residents, but also for many clinicians in the hospital. CT viewboxes are relatively cloistered, insulating the work of radiologists from patients and non-medical laity – but open to clinical colleagues. Clinicians of various sorts in the hospital make periodic pilgrimages to the viewbox to view 'original' films and to confer with radiologists. Viewboxes thus serve as ritual centres, and the films displayed on them retain a kind of 'cult value', deriving from their originality and the regulation of their handling and viewing.[7]

Physician-at-viewbox has for decades been a prominent formula in the popular iconography of doctoring. In teaching hospitals particularly, but also in non-teaching hospitals, the viewbox has served a special role in situating performances of group *autopsis.* Autopsis: seeing for oneself, of course, but also, in its oldest connotations, rhetorics of testimony: saying what one sees (Pagden 1993).

Each viewbox – or 'board' – offers four panels (14"×17") of backlighting, with a motorised mechanism to allow rapid scrolling through many films. The board's contiguous layout of writing surface, logbook, telephone, dictation machine, footpedals, and folder slots, is calculated to optimise workflow.[8] Mechanised viewboxes were originally developed to facilitate large-volume radiological review, and they became essential with the advent of CT scanners, which generate ever-increasing numbers of slices per study.

Handwork

Diagnosis at the viewbox, and in the conference room, hinges on a great deal of handwork. Manual practices of 'hanging films', scrolling through studies on the viewbox, using the dictaphone, writing while speaking on the phone, shuffling films and papers while chewing: such practices define chains of evidential custody, mark territories among cases, exemplify dexterity. Sometimes they define hierarchies – as when an attending hands off stacks of film for the resident to hang, or hands a scrawled reference to a student to retrieve from the library. Some handwork is described in scripts and protocols – how long before a CT-guided biopsy one must summon the pathologist; how to reboot the MagicView system. Some is learned by emulation, imitation, and embodied as habit. Some rules are written to break, or remake, habits. 'No gloves!' says the sign at the scanner room phone. Many of these practices are constitutive, not epiphenomenal, in the project of knowledge making.

One of these skills – 'hanging films' – is worth further consideration. The radiologist (or trainee) whose hands are swift and sure in moving films from folder to board is like a skilful card dealer. Film-handling skill is non-trivial in distinguishing her from clinical colleagues. Such skill comprises: knowing where to look on the film for patient-identifying data; knowing how to correlate the last slice on one panel with the first slice of another; swiftly recognising left and right, forward and backward; knowing guild conventions for 'mounting' – old study left of new, non-contrast before contrast, soft tissues windows separate from bone. But it also involves gestural knowledge – how to push a floppy film through the air with the fingers and slip it beneath the monofilament retainer on the board – or how to slip in a small stack and spread it out with one sweep of the hands (Figure 7.3).

In the reading room, a fellow tells a colleague on the phone what has delayed him in delivering some films. He explains that he is speaking around a piece of hard candy. 'The [infectious disease] team came down and gave me one ... I put up about twenty thousand films in about thirty seconds and they gave me one ... There was about fifty thousand of them – a whole flock – I didn't think the room could hold them all.' His intellectual contributions to a patient's diagnosis are entirely elided from this workshop tale of expert handling of film and colleagues' bodies.

A range of manual practices inflects viewbox enterprises of reading – twined in various ways with speech. Postures (e.g., sitting, with composure, sometimes with eager lean), gestures (e.g., pointing), locutions (e.g., formulae for dictating official reports) proper to diagnostic work are learned and propagated in small social groupings. Many of these 'body techniques' are learned by example and imitation, or trial and correction, and perfected with practice. Some of them are skills which must be learned and demonstrated before they can be discarded: for example, attendings are often spared by underlings from the chore of hanging films; and in dictation of formal reports, attendings are permitted to omit much detail that residents are obliged to include.

Interpretive Craft

The radiological craft practice I wish to forefront here, as a privileged focus of apprenticeship-style teaching, is a rather more cognitive one (which is not to say it is disembodied). This is the 'abductive' part of diagnosis. It belongs to the ethos of tracking and hunting which I suggested might be one echo of the term 'suite'—and is associated with theatrical devices of intrigue introduced above. *Abduction* is a philosopher's, not a radiologist's, locution: it is Charles Peirce's term for a modality of reason that others have variously called conjecture, hypothesis, ratiocination, even analysis – not so much new with Peirce as newly distinguished from, and restored to parity with, its more familiar cousins, deduction and induction.[9]

In Peirce's typology, abduction stretches across the same cognitive elements as do deduction and induction, but in a different order, and with different effects. Abduction's product is, in Peirce's terminology, a 'case' – some causal or situational arrangement that plausibly connects particular observed facts with received general 'rules'. Abduction's connection of facts to rules, findings to givens, is conjectural and perhaps hazardous: the abduced case is judged according to criteria of 'fit' or 'satisfactoriness'.

Abduction thus summons, and manifests, forms of aesthetic engagement. It is folded into the economy of intrigue in the diagnostic enterprise, which includes suites of affect: puzzlement, frustration, astonishment, admiration, etc. Such are the aesthetic effects conjured up by detective stories – and these are the literary matrix in which, indeed, much of the secondary literature on abduction has been produced (Eco and Sebeok 1983). The viewbox is a privileged site of exchange in this economy of intrigue. It is a stage for abductive theater.

To speak of intrigue or abduction as theatre, or as economy, is to forefront their social and cultural dimensions – i.e. to resist their assimilation to private cognition or affect, or to the constitution of Nature's puzzle, or natural curiosity. Silent puzzlement or private abduction are no doubt possible; 'nature' surely presents mysteries; but at the viewbox, and throughout the diagnostic enterprise, skills of tracking disease are learned and practised in groups, in an ethos of culprit-pursuit. These theatre-groups are stratified according to hierarchies of training, and divided by disciplinary expertise – and both the hierarchies and specialisation inform, just as they are propagated and revised by, performances of abductive craft.

I want to characterise very briefly the way in which radiological work is abductive. And, my claims about affect aside, I want to note how quick and automatic abduction can be. I will then consider felicity conditions for associations of abductive craft with thicker kinds of intrigue.

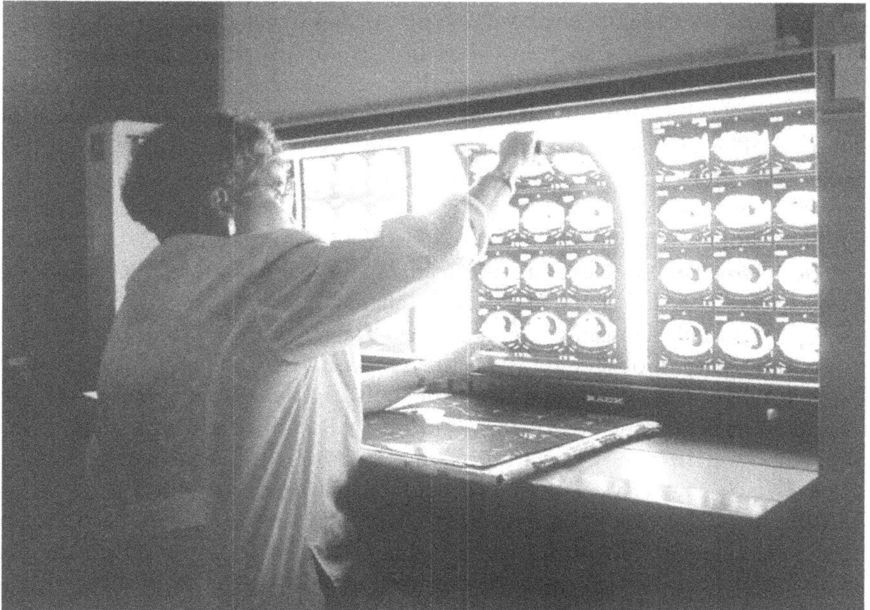

Figure 7.3 *Hanging films.*

Peirce's analysis of abduction uses terminology quite suited to consideration of the work of radiologists. Particular facts, handled in light of certain general rules, may permit one to abduce a case. Radiologists don't call them facts, but they do speak of 'findings'. This is the term which heads the first, descriptive section of the formal X-ray report.

Radiological findings are marks, clues, traces. In practice they must first be distinguished from 'artefacts' – traces of technological glitch rather than bodily structure. Risk of confusing findings with artefacts requires constant vigilance. Findings are then described – with just enough detail to facilitate comparison with findings on other scans, findings in the grand archive. Probably the first schema of sorting findings is that of normal/abnormal. 'Make friends with the normal' is an oft-repeated maxim about preparation to recognise findings. Expectations of normal findings structure one's review of a scan. For example, the litany of a mental checklist – 'adrenal pancreas spleen kidneys within normal limits' – can offer a kind of comfort, constitute a series of nods to friends; it exemplifies relations among norms, memory, expectation and rhythms of habit. (Trainees' dictations are longer than attendings', in part because of their repetition – for the benefit of overseers as well as their own senses of security – of such formulaic lists.) That findings can be friends reminds us that percepts are not morally or aesthetically neutral: evaluative qualifiers are common, in the conference room and at the viewbox: 'an exquisite demonstration', or 'an ugly [i.e., malignant] kind of [contrast-] enhancement'. (See Grasseni's comments in the Introduction to this volume on ethics of perception.)

On the other side of the abductive process are what Peirce called 'general rules'. There are many such in CT radiology. Brains shrink as patients age. Breast cancer metastasises to lung and bone. Contrast shows up in arteries before veins. The most common mediastinal tumour after the fifth decade of life is ... The radiologist's (or trainee's) command of general rules, distilled from 'the literature' and his own cumulative knowledge, structures his handling of findings.

These ingredients, findings and rules condition abductive work. From them, between them, cases are abduced: 'I think this patient has interstitial lung disease', or, 'Looks like he's failing chemo'.

In Peircean abduction, the gap between the generality of known rules and the particularity of observed facts is filled by conjecture. This gap is narrowed considerably if general rules are especially particularised, or if facts are especially typical. The 'fit' of the abduced case is more automatic, its status more certain, that is, when findings are so typical that there is already a general rule that covers them. In such a situation, in which the case is thoroughly determined, or overdetermined, by the pincer-grip of rules on findings, it is said that findings 'are diagnostic'. In such a circumstance, abducing the case is reduced to 'pattern-recognition'. Though maintaining a sufficiently robust repertoire of general rules can be challenging to a radiologist, such effective reduction of her craft to rule-following is also less 'fun'. This is particularly a concern for readers of CT scans – as suggested in these reflections of one senior radiologist:

> I enjoy the diagnostic process, the intrigue, the curiosity, the satisfaction of search, or not ... Anyway, I tell my residents, and they look at me askance – fuddy-duddy old fart – I say 'CT makes it too damn easy for you'. It makes it too damn easy. You can see things sitting right there. You got a 3 mm slice and got this darn mass there you know ...
>
> ... Because the modern medical student and house officer is in a hurry and they want the answer and the slice is right there, there's the answer right there. Whereas the beauty of radiology, to me anyway – maybe because again I come from a different tradition – has been the curiosity and the question – the curiosity has been piqued by the subtle findings. I tell the residents, you know, I like to be able to explain everything on this plain film. And if I see a problem and I can't figure out why it is, I'll feel like I've been frustrated. I like to be able to look at this and understand everything that's going on. If I have to use CT to help me, fine. But most of the time, I can sort of get a sense of what's going on without that ... And it's the fun of that. Which is really exciting to me.

Radiology is extraordinarily self-conscious about its own cognitive processes, as well as its logistics of perception. On the one hand, it strives for certainty, towards an ideal of total legibility, instant and unambiguous recognisability and classifiability of the culprit morphologies it pursues. On the other hand, it not only understands, but folds into its pedagogical rituals, the frequent ambiguity of seeing, the trickiness of lesions, the provisional status of some so-called rules. It actively produces diagnostic intrigue in some of its favoured teaching rituals. Trainees like the challenge of puzzling cases.

Thus a favoured genre in radiology journals, teaching conferences, and in continuing education web sites (e.g., AuntMinnie.com, a 'resident-friendly' web site), is the puzzling unknown case. In such a case, the findings are usually *not* straightforwardly 'diagnostic'; the clinical contexts given are limited, insufficient to determine a proper answer. The resident's diagnostic efforts are necessarily provisional, conjectural; they have the status of a hazarded guess – informed, but not certain. If she is right, she may enjoy a moment of delight and pride; if wrong, she feels chastened, and retreats to amend her descriptions of findings, or the inadequacy of her repertoires of rules.

The puzzling case – as presented in a teaching conference or in the pages of a trade journal – is understood to be something of a contrivance. As noted above, quite often something is withheld – key facts, suggestive clinical circumstances. Or, something might be added, such as conflicting evidence. Or the case has been chosen because of its atypicality. Radiologists and trainees develop and engage such puzzling cases as theatrical props, and make no apologies for the artifice or obfuscation that is often ingredient in them.[11]

A senior radiologist is attending *du jour* on Body CT service. On the viewbox is a study with a familiar name – from a previous encounter, three years earlier. The team is caught up with work, and the attending is in an expansive mood. He puts up several of the old films and begins to tell the tale of their first reading, at the time of the first 'presentation' of this patient to CT.

> CT Resident: Is this a true history?
> CT Attending: Yeah.
> Resident: All right.
> Attending: I would not pull your leg. Everything I say is nothing but honest truth. That's the reason I'm trying to teach you here, is to be confident, instead of 'maybe this, maybe that' …

The attending points to an image showing a mass in the inferior vena cava, a trunk vein. There is contrast around it but the mass itself does not take up contrast.

> Attending: The history of this case comes in such a way that obviously everybody saw the big IVC … And so they thought that it was a clot. And [*filmflap*] what do you think. How about just a bland clot?
> Resident: I wouldn't expect it to expand the lumen.
> Attending: OK. I agree …

The expanded vessel is more like something cancer would do. Therefore the clinicians biopsied the lesion. No cancer.

> Resident: So they biopsied this thing and it came back negative.
> Attending: Yeah. Negative. And then what would you say?
> Resident: Ah, I'd say, it could be sampling error.
> Attending: So that's the reason we did the CT like this. [*filmflap*]
> Resident: OK.
> Attending: And we even did MR.
> Resident: And MR I bet showed enhancement of the mass.
> Attending: Ah, no more than this.
> Resident: OK.
> Attending: Like this. And then we saw these. So what do you think?

The second CT is a high-resolution study. It is now possible to see dots of white in the mass. These could be contrast or something else dense.

> Attending: I'm just telling you the story as I saw them three years ago. As it unfolded.
> Resident: The question would be checking on your pre-contrast making sure it's not anything like calcium.
> Attending: No calcium, excellent idea.
> Resident: If it is contrast, it's either a tumor …
> Attending: Mm-hmm.
> Resident: Or collaterals.
> Attending: Collaterals. What do you mean by collaterals? …

Resident:	Um.
Attending:	That's the question. What are they, these white dots there?
Resident:	I think it's probably neovascularization inside the tumor.
Attending:	OK, that's one possibility; there's another possibility if it's a bland clot. ...
Resident:	That it was – that it was recanalization.
Attending:	Exactly. That's the only two possibilities ... It could be a neovascularity as you say, or if it's a bland clot it could be a recanalization.

After posing the dilemma – cancer or bland clot? – and while waiting for an answer, which is not immediately forthcoming from the resident, the attending raises the stakes. Is this something that should be biopsied? Excised? Irradiated? (if cancer) –or merely treated with blood thinner? (if clot). He moves the tale into the present tense when he does this. He taps on the film with his pointer. To the resident: What are you going to tell this patient? Dramatic pause: urgency of an imagined decisional present. But then he moves his tale back to the past tense, and another device of heightening suspense. It makes sense that the resident is stumped. Back then, the radiologists and the clinicians were all stumped too. They did not know what to do with the patient, other than admit her to the hospital 'for more tests'.

In this telling, the sun set on the indecision and confusion of the combined clinicians and radiologists. The attending went home:

> ... I said, I think it's tumor, just as you said, expansion, everything else, but I really can't tell if this is recanalization or if it's arterial neovascularity. And I drove home and I was eating dinner, and a thought came to me ... [T]hat was early in the evening, it was like 7–8 o'clock in the evening.

It came to him. The patient had cancer. With pride and elation at making the diagnosis – tempered with concern for the patient, he hastened to add – he called the patient's clinical attending, also at home, and relayed his conclusion. In the absence of the images he did not explain. When asked how sure he was that this was cancer and not bland clot, he replied: 'If this is not cancer, I will eat the film.'

'I am not a betting man', says the attending to the resident. 'What made me so sure that this was cancer? It is in the picture.'

More silence. 'Want me to tell you?' 'No!' says the resident. 'Give me some time to think.' He is engaged and vexed. The attending revisits the tale and dots the *i*'s. No longer a question of cancer or clot, but: how did I know that this was cancer, and not clot? Still no answer. Give up? No!

The CT fellow returns to the room – prompting another, briefer, spinning of the tale. The fellow is puzzled too. A gratifying moment for the attending. But time is wasting.

The attending has spoken only the words 'the arteries' when the fellow hastens to blurt the answer. (The resident has lost his chance.)

Why, the contrast is in the arterial phase! From looking at other vessels it can be seen that the scanner cut through this level while the flush of contrast was still mostly in arteries, and not much in veins, as yet. In this lesion, to be able to say that the blush of contrast was in feeder arteries, rather than in venous canals, made for the key distinction between tumour and clot.

Attending: That's what it is, it's in the arterial phase.
Fellow: Cool.
Attending: I said 'no way'. So I told him, I said, 'I'll eat the film if this is not cancer.'
Resident: And he was happy with that?
Attending: He thought that I was so good. He'd never forget that I – that's why we have a standing joke that [this is] my private patient ... It was all logic, nothing fancy. [*filmflap*]

The resident is embarrassed but quick to signal understanding. He turns to the fat file in his lap, and notes that the patient had also undergone other studies. 'May I look at her venogram?', he asks. 'You can look at anything you want', says the attending. Leaning back, he returns pointer to pocket, quite satisfied.

This attending's tale is one of an interpretive subtlety overlooked by many, and his own late-breaking insight. All assimilable to the good of the patient. He tells it, he says, like it happened. One suspects he also tells it like he has told it before. The present intrigue of this case is produced by narrative devices, tactical withholdings, whose relation to the primal contexts of diagnosis is historical and mimetic. This retelling is thus much like case narratives of the conference room: it is founded on old images, in a pedagogical interlude – and it places a resident in an interrogative situation that simulates the difficulties of primary diagnosis. The resident is challenged to assume a position and exercise faculties which cannot be taught by rote or rule: he is challenged to make an abductive leap – akin to making a judgement.

The tissue proved nothing in this case: pathology was less a 'gold standard' then a red herring. 'Sampling error', the resident suggested – granting room for Nature to remain true to itself. Proof here hinged on timing of contrast delivery. For all the initial confusion and the stumping of the resident, this was not an arcane case: finessing contrast logistics has become a bread-and-butter issue for radiologists.

This intrigue took shape as expressly pedagogical contrivance; the exchanges it rehearses, however, once unfolded organically, as it were, were within shopfloor discourse. They were typical of other exchanges in radiological work at the viewbox in the late 1990s – where comings and goings of clinical colleagues served to extend and ravel a knot of intrigue around many cases. Viewbox rituals were no less theatrical than formal teaching conferences; but the incompleteness of clinical suspicions, the contradictoriness of non-radiological data introduced, the clever competitiveness of interspecialty colloquy, served to thicken diagnostic plots and summon the suite of affective engagements I have glossed as intrigue. Sometimes, often, radiologists found themselves in the role of clarifying a preceding mystery (one they had no idea existed outside the reading room); on other occasions they assumed roles of witnesses whose testimony was contested, cross-examined. In either way, radiologists felt involved as intrigants, effectively, in generating, supporting, or consummating adventurous exercises of abductive craft.

This improvisational theatre of intrigue at the viewbox accomplished two things. It exemplified for all participants how the radiological diagnostic economy (whose indices are typically quantified and objectified as throughput, reporting time, error) called for irreducibly qualitative exercises of crafty acumen and associated forms of aesthetic engagement – on the shopfloor, not merely in formal educational exercises. The second thing was to engage radiological trainees first-hand in the observation, emulation and practice of this abductive craft in, so to speak, 'real life'.

I emphasise the importance of this last aspect, namely, the emulation of abduction. What I have called the 'aesthetic' dimension of abductive thinking – the judgement of 'fit' between particular findings and general rules – is something that cannot be taught propositionally. This is akin to the Kantian observation about judgement, that it cannot be presented through concepts, but requires exhibition – *Darstellung* (Kant 1987, 80 (§17:233)). Edgar Poe noted something like this as well at the outset of his inaugural detective story, *The Murders in the Rue Morgue*: 'The mental features discoursed of as the analytical are, in themselves, but little susceptible of analysis. We appreciate them only in their effects' (Poe 1978, 527–28.)[12]

Disappearance of the Mechanical Viewbox

I began this chapter by remarking on the virtues of the hospital's indigenous term 'suite' as an ethnographic trope, referring not only to rooms but to practices of following. But recently, on returning to scenes of my original fieldwork, I discovered another register of 'following' – one whose rapidity has surprised me. Many of the practices that I observed so meticulously have already disappeared. The CT suite has changed radically in just a few years. Forms of handwork so recently constitutive of diagnostic truthmaking turn out to have been elided, eclipsed – and with astonishing speed.

The big change is that, across radiology, especially in CT, film is disappearing – indeed, already gone, from University Hospital, except for films sent in from some 'outside hospitals'. Without film, no more chemical wetcraft or darkroom film-handling chores, no more massive film management and storage enterprise, no more 'sneaker-net' of film couriers. Most important, in the reading room, no more mechanical film viewbox. A PACS (picture archiving and communications system) has replaced the viewbox. The image display workstation in the reading room now is much tidier, and because there are others like it distributed throughout the hospital, images in the reading room no longer claim the status of 'originals'.

The disappearance of the mechanical viewbox – conveyor belt for a bygone day's X-ray docket – summons little nostalgia from radiologists. They are glad now to scroll through phosphor screens rather than toggle a noisy film procession, glad for 'stacked' slices rather than gridded slices, glad for easier reproduction of studies for teaching and research. Throughput is faster, reporting is faster – all to the good, since case volume has close to doubled in the last five years.

Back and forth the films used to go on that viewbox, or round and round, each study referenced multiple times, until the docket of studies had been read and overread, up and down the radiological hierarchy and often across several specialties. What a lot of traffic that was through the reading room, pilgrim clinicians and their trainees, all migrating to the central viewbox to see and discuss original films. CT radiologists used to find their work-flow interrupted all the time. Yet you could also say that the viewbox in the reading room was, as one old-timer put it, the axle of the wheel.

Is it possible that the demise of the mechanical viewbox, as a ritual centre of diagnostic work, may diminish opportunities for social propagation of diagnostic intrigues, and for the stimulus these afford to emulative learning of abductive craft? Might diminished face-to-face engagement with clinical colleagues diminish the richness of pedagogical role-playing – clinicians instructing radiologists, radiologists instructing clinicians? Perhaps the reduced interruption of radiological viewing results in more elaborated forms of viewbox teaching, more intense apprentice relations, within the radiological hierarchy itself. To be sure, there are plenty of occasions in the reading rooms today, in less-interrupted work at tidier workstations, when trainees can register astonishment and admiration in the face of some diagnostic feat, or be gently corrected in their own efforts. (There are also forms of apprenticeship that invert the political hierarchy: residents, who have generally been more adept than attendings in assimilation of new digital tools, often find themselves in the role of tutor in PACS-craft.) There is still the telephone, which supports surprising amounts of cross-disciplinary colloquy. And there are still interspecialty performances of skilled visioning elsewhere in the hospital, in conferences and at the various distributed workstations where PACS images are reviewed. But the radiology reading room itself has become just a bit more factory-like, more beholden to Taylorist logics of efficient throughput. And the pedagogical implications of these changes in interprofessional colloquy have not yet been examined in the medical literature.

Do these observations betray simple nostalgia? Do they constitute yet another instance of the Weberian critique of progressive disenchantment by instrumental rationality (Weber 1952)? Perhaps aspects of diagnosis will remain enchanted projects, like divination for the ancients. But specific discursive forms and 'cognitive artefacts' – like the rise of the detective story in the nineteenth century – play crucial historical roles. In any case we are reminded that curiosity, imagination, judgement are best thought of not as innate faculties or private virtues that the worker brings to the workplace, but as faculties produced and reproduced in social settings, through suites of cultured practice – and thus worthy of careful consideration, as regards which ritual and pedagogical conditions will best encourage their flourishing. What is called for, of course – as in so many cases when ethnographic analysis encounters historical forces, including rapidly changing technologies – is further ethnographic engagement, in new configurations of cultural practice.

Notes

1 This chapter is based on ethnographic fieldwork in US hospitals in the late 1990s, and distilled from analyses developed at greater length in my book, *CT Suite* (Duke University Press, forthcoming). Medical imaging craftwork discussed here is clinical/diagnostic, to be distinguished from imaging research considered by Cohn and Roepstorff in their essays in this volume.

2 There are many suites of personage and practice that this account elides. Technologists, nurses, clerks and others are discussed in my book in their relations to radiological diagnostic practice. On CT techs in particular, at a historical juncture when there was much more interaction with radiologists about work with the scanner apparatus, see Barley (1984).

3 My welcome in this suite as ethnographer, to follow along after my own fashion, ask questions, take notes, and make audiotapes of 'shoptalk' – as well as my capacity to understand what I heard and saw – was in various ways predicated upon prior training and status as an internal medicine physician, i.e. a member of an affine guild. I was seen and treated at times as an apprentice. But I also preserved prerogatives of the stranger, one whose objectivity is, in Simmel's (1950) terms, an amalgam of 'distance and nearness, indifference and involvement' (on this theme, see Grasseni's introduction to this volume). Even when assuming postures of the apprentice, I remained a '*potential* wanderer'—one who could 'not quite overcome the freedom of coming and going' (Simmel 1950, 402).

4 US residency programmes in diagnostic radiology, as described in a central database maintained by the AMA (American Medical Association), may or may not have 'formal mentorship programs' – but all support mentorship in various ways.

5 Here I mean subspecialisation on various levels, in and out of radiology. CT, a technology dedicated to non-invasive slicing of bodies, has also sliced up hospital space and culture. (This claim cannot be unpacked within this essay.)

6 There are various ways in which reading CT scans differs from, or constitutes a subspecialty within, radiological reading more generally. Perhaps the most significant difference derives from the need in CT reading to integrate successive slices into a sense of volume.

7 'Original' films have special status even in CT, notwithstanding the fact that images are derived from digital datasets. On cult value, cf. Benjamin (1969). Cult value here stands in contrast with 'exhibition value' (as Marxian 'use value' is contrasted with 'exchange value').

8 On historical development of radiological recordkeeping in service to managerial concerns, see Howell (1995).

9 See Peirce 1940 and 1957 for a useful sample from the still-scattered Peircean dossier on abduction.

10 This term has pejorative connotations for radiologists seeking to forefront the importance of their judgement; but in other areas where it is used more systematically – notably, by computer programmers in artificial intelligence (AI) fields – it signifies quite complex

processes. On nuances of pattern recognition from the perspective of natural historians, see: Pantin (1954, cited in Polanyi 1962); Law and Lynch (1990).

11 Puzzling cases, both in their making and their solving, constitute a form of serious professional play – thus are analogous in this diagnostic culture to forms of play discussed by Cohn in experiments with brain images, and by Grasseni in uses of figurines in learning bovine connoisseurship, in essays in this volume.

12 Abduction in detective work also prototypically draws upon the body of the detective (another story). See Harrowitz, 'The Body of the Detective Model', in Eco and Sebeok (1983). Relations of gestural knowledge with 'low sciences' of artisan cultures and with the rise of metrology and standards are discussed by Schaffer in a fine historical case study (1997). Embodied and other aspects of cunning and crafty knowing, including their engagement in agonistic contexts, are developed in discussions of *metis* – to be distinguished from *theoreia* and *episteme* – in Detienne and Vernant (1991). My understandings of modes of craft-knowledge have benefited greatly from exchanges with J. Farquhar (1993) and R. Tyson (1988).

References

Barley, S. 1984. *The Professional, the Semi-Professional, and the Machine*. Cambridge, Mass.: MIT (dissertation).

Benjamin, W. 1969. 'The Work of Art in the Age of Mechanical Reproduction', in *Illuminations*, trans. H. Zohn, ed. H. Arendt. New York: Schocken Books, 223–26.

Detienne, M., and J. Vernant, 1991. *Cunning Intelligence in Greek Culture and Society*, trans. Lloyd. Chicago: University of Chicago Press.

Eco, U., and T. Sebeok, 1983. *The Sign of Three: Dupin, Holmes, Peirce*. Bloomington: Indiana University Press.

Eddy, D. and C. Clanton, 1982. 'The Art of Diagnosis: Solving the Clinicopathological Exercise', *New England Journal of Medicine* 308 (21): 1263–68.

Farquhar, J. 1993. *Knowing Practice: The Clinical Encounter of Chinese Medicine*. Boulder: Westview Press.

Ginzburg, C. 1989. 'Clues: Roots of an Evidential Paradigm', in *Clues, Myths, and the Historical Method*, trans. J. Tedeschi and A. Tedeschi. Baltimore: Johns Hopkins University Press, 96–125.

Howell, J. 1995. *Technology in the Hospital: Transforming Patient Care in the Early Twentieth Century*. Baltimore: Johns Hopkins University Press.

Hunter, K. 1991. 'The Representation of the Patient', in *Doctors' Stories*. Princeton: Princeton University Press.

Kant, I. 1987. *The Critique of Judgment*, trans. Pluhar. Indianapolis: Hackett.

Law, J. and M. Lynch, 1990. 'Lists, Field Guides, and the Descriptive Organization of Seeing: Birdwatching as an Exemplary Observational Activity', in *Representation in Scientific Practice*, eds. M. Lynch and S. Woolgar, Cambridge, Mass.: MIT Press, 267–99.

Pagden, A. 1993. 'The Autoptic Imagination', in *European Encounters with the New World*. New Haven: Yale University Press.

Pantin, C. 1954. 'The Recognition of Species', *Science Progress* 42.

Peirce, C. 1940. 'Abduction and Induction', in *The Philosophy of Charles Peirce*, ed. J. Buchler. London: Routledge & Kegan Paul, 150–56.

Peirce, C. 1957. 'Deduction, Induction, and Hypothesis' and '[The Logic of Abduction]', in *Charles S. Peirce*, ed. V. Tomas. New York: Liberal Arts Press, 125–43, 235–55.

Poe, E. 1978. 'The Murders in the Rue Morgue', in T. Mabbott, ed., *Collected Works of Edgar Allan Poe*, vol. II. Cambridge, Mass.: Harvard University Press.

Polanyi, M. 1962. *Personal Knowledge: Towards a Post-Critical Philosophy*. Chicago: University of Chicago Press.

Schaffer, S. 1997. 'Experimenters' Techniques, Dyers' Hands, and the Electric Planetarium', *Isis* 88 (3): 456–83.

Simmel, G. 1950. 'The Stranger', in *The Sociology of Georg Simmel*, trans. K. Wolff. Glencoe, IL: The Free Press, 802–08.

Tyson, R. 1988. 'Odysseus and the Cyclops' (unpublished essay).

Weber, M. 1952. 'Science as a Vocation', in *From Max Weber*, trans. and ed. H. Gerth and C. Mills. London: Routledge & Kegan Paul, 129–56.

Chapter 8

Training the Naturalist's Eye in the Eighteenth Century: Perfect Global Visions and Local Blind Spots

Daniela Bleichmar

In an age that identified vision as the means to investigate and understand nature, perhaps the worst tragedy that could befall a naturalist was to lose his eyesight. This was the unfortunate condition of Georg Everhard Rumphius (1627–1702), a German doctor, naturalist and collector living in the Moluccas in the employment of the Dutch East India Company. Despite this considerable challenge, over the second half of the seventeenth century Rumphius amassed an incomparable collection of natural objects, many of which he sold to the Grand Duke of Tuscany as the basis of an impressive natural history cabinet. Rumphius also had many items drawn, and wrote or dictated their scientific descriptions in preparation for publication. These images and texts furnished the material for two titles appearing posthumously over the first half of the eighteenth century, *The Ambonese Curiosity Cabinet* (1705) and *The Ambonese Herbarium* (1741–55). Both works included the same portrait of Rumphius (Figure 8.1).

The engraving shows Rumphius, aged sixty-eight, sitting at a work table crowded with plants, shells and books. Corals and other natural marine products fill the shelf on the wall behind him, while two specimens are suspended with string from nails on the wall. In the foreground, in the lower left corner, a book or notebook is open to a page showing the image of a plant, while the facing page is used to name the authors of the drawing and the engraving. Unable to see the objects on the table, the naturalist fixes his vacant gaze outside the frame of the image and uses his hands to examine the objects on the table. His serious face is tense with concentration as his hand

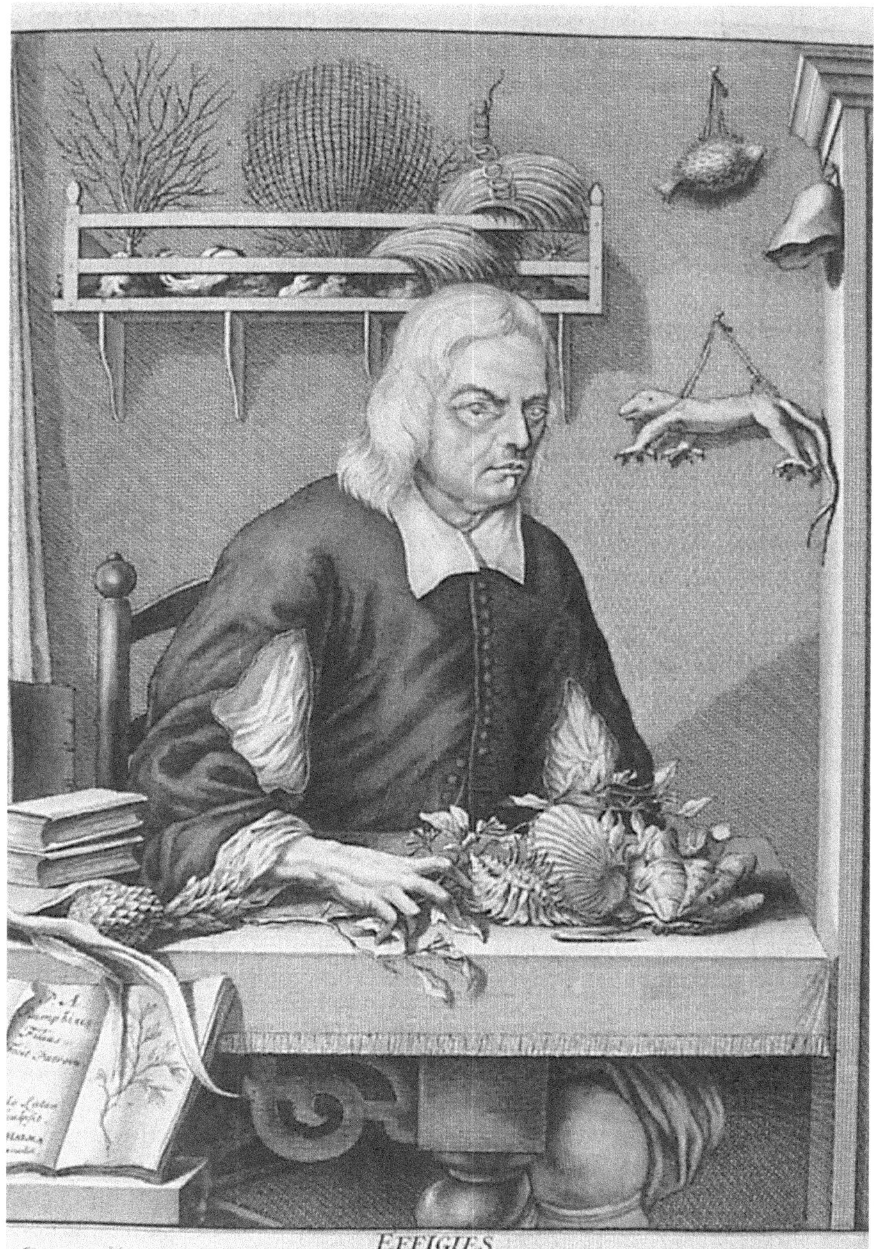

Figure 8.1 Portrait of Georg Everhard Rumphius. Frontmatter of his *De Amboinsche rariteitkamer* (Amsterdam, 1705). (Courtesy of the Linnean Society of London)

actively and forcefully investigates the objects it holds. This, clearly, is not a depiction of an invalid but a portrait of a naturalist at work. The Latin encomium underneath the portrait proclaims: 'Though he be blind, his mental eyes are so sharp that no one can best him at inquiry or discernment. Rumphius is German by birth but his loyalty and pen are completely Dutch. Let the work say the rest' (Rumphius 1999).

The paradoxical portrait of the blind naturalist with incomparable eyesight encapsulates three related ideas that I examine in this essay. First, naturalists considered visual skill the defining trait of their practice and the basis of their method. Collecting and classifying, the twin obsessions of eighteenth-century natural history, were predicated on the ability of the trained eye to assess, possess and order. Nature was investigated through sight, and the eye provided the instrument with which to approach the world as well as the means to discipline it. The investigation of nature depended upon the analysis of visual information, and the naturalist was defined first and foremost as an observer. For this reason, the process of becoming a naturalist revolved around visual training. Naturalists' notion of sight went beyond the physiological act of seeing to involve an expert type of viewing that involved training and specialised practices of observation and representation – not merely sight but rather insight.

Second, Rumphius's portrait reminds us that natural history was not only a visually oriented practice but also one that relied heavily on material culture. If the eye was the consummate tool of the eighteenth-century naturalist, the botanical eye was an extremely active creature, in constant motion among drawn or engraved images, specimens in collections, and textual information in manuscript or print. Illustrated books were particularly important to eighteenth-century naturalists, who valued their libraries as much as their specimen collections.[1] As I will describe in this essay, books standardised methods for collecting and collating material and established shared guidelines for observing, describing, naming, classifying and representing. In this way, books provided a visual and verbal vocabulary that was shared by naturalists throughout and beyond Europe. They provided standards against which naturalists could gauge the value of their own work, as well as models for them to emulate or react against. Thus, books helped to define and arbitrate a community of competent and relevant reader-practitioners.[2] Books also served to demarcate what naturalists actually needed to do in the field, namely, to describe any local productions not included within the European printed inventory of global nature, to rectify any discrepancies, and to resolve incomplete or erroneous descriptions.

Furthermore, printed books provided naturalists with the illustrations they needed to approach nature, with parameters for producing new images, and with a medium for presenting their own contributions to natural history. Printed illustrations allowed travellers to ascertain whether the plants and animals they encountered were truly unknown, in which case they could be introduced into the literature and linked to their discoverer's name – ideally, accompanied by an image. In the eighteenth century, images provided an entry point into the exploration of nature, functioned as a key instrument for producing knowledge, and constituted the foremost result of natural investigations. Images operated at every point of a trajectory that moved from the collection of natural data to its incorporation into a global inventory of nature through textual description and visual representation.

Third, the engraving intimates that the visual and material aspects of natural history were inextricably linked to European colonialism and global trade. Rumphius accumulated his remarkable collection of natural specimens in the Moluccas, and this provenance mattered to readers of the books that catalogued that collection. Although the ways in which European naturalists and collectors understood natural specimens and nature as a whole changed greatly throughout the early modern period, a constant remained throughout: a predilection for naturalia from distant lands. The reasons for this interest went beyond exoticism, although this was certainly a factor. The collection – of objects, images or textual descriptions – ideally functioned as a microcosm representative of the whole world, whether natural objects formed part of sixteenth- and seventeenth-century *Wunderkammern* or existed within the ordered cabinets of the eighteenth-century taxonomist who attempted to compile an exhaustive catalogue of nature.[3] Naturalists and collectors, authors and readers, all considered travel, natural history and the exploration of distant and exotic lands to be integrally connected. The French naturalist Michel Adanson, for instance, combined in a single book his descriptions of Senegalese shells with an account of his travels through the region. The book's title is *Natural History of Senegal. Shells*; its subtitle, *With an Abbreviated Relation of a Voyage to This Country in the Years 1749–1753*. In the Preface to the second section, Adanson anthropomorphised shells and presented conchology as ethnographic travel literature. He wrote,

> If we examine attentively this new and entirely forgotten population [shells], if we consider in particular each of the beings that compose it, we will discover in their customs, in their actions, in their movements, in their way of life, an infinity of very curious things, of interesting facts capable of capturing the attention of the avid and intelligent observer. (Adanson 1757: x)[4]

In this way, Adanson drew explicit connections between the act of observing, the naturalist's persona as a capable observer, the study of natural history and the experience of travel. These associations were evident to other authors. For the French pharmacist Fusée Aublet, the most significant problem with European knowledge of American flora in the late 1750s was that the majority of available textual descriptions and images were inaccurate or incomplete. Naturalists, he urged, desperately needed more exact and complete descriptions and figures, and for these they depended on travellers who could observe, describe and illustrate accurately and appropriately (Aublet 1775: xxvi). As Pierre André de Latreille made clear in his continuation to Buffon's *Histoire naturelle, générale et particuliere,* not every traveller was capable of providing the type of results that would prove useful to naturalists. He explained,

> I admire the courage of those travellers who, to enlarge our collections, brave the furies of the vast Ocean, and face a thousand dangers to collect ... rare or unknown plants and animals. But I think that zoology would gain more if skilled observers spread throughout different regions of the world studied, at great length and over many years, the natural riches [of those regions]. (Latreille 1802–5, vol. 1: 61)[5]

Skilled ways of seeing served as a mechanism for identifying, translating, transporting, and ultimately appropriating nature.

Training the Naturalist's Eye: Visual Culture in Eighteenth-century Natural History

Carl Linnaeus's *Systema Naturae* (1735), one of the central works of the eighteenth-century taxonomical turn, proposed not only a system but also a concomitant work procedure based on specialised techniques of observation. The *Systema* presented tables outlining a taxonomy of the vegetal, animal and mineral kingdom. A separate chart provided Linnaeus's sexual system of botanical classification, guiding the reader step by step through the process of determining to which one of twenty-four classes any given plant belonged. The process consisted of posing a standard series of set yes-or-no questions, with each answer eliminating certain choices until one arrived at the plant's classification.[6] Linnaeus was proposing not only a taxonomy but also a methodology based on observation, a point made even more clearly a year later when the twenty-four classes were depicted pictorially by the great botanical illustrator Georg Dyonisius Ehret (Figure 8.2).[7]

Ehret's table includes twenty-four figures, one representing the distinguishing traits of each of the Linnaean plant classes, which are characterised by the structure of the flower and seed. Figure A represents the first class, *monandria,* characterised by having one stamen; figure B shows the second class, *diandria,* with two stamens; figure F the sixth, *hexandria,* with six stamens, and so on with various combinations of stamens and pistils.[8] The table was reproduced or adapted in countless botanical books of the time, and contributed greatly to the popularity of Linnaean classification, making it appear simple, direct and seemingly foolproof. The shift from chart to table offered a different representational technique as well as a move towards making methodology invisible. By eclipsing the interrogation procedure, it suggested that the Linnaean system provided an immediate taxonomy based exclusively on sight, without the need for logical analysis. In order to classify a plant, it promised, the botanist needed simply to look at a flower, count its stamens and pistils, and note their structural arrangement. The chart transported theory out of the page, internalising it within the eyes of the naturalist.

Linnaeus's *Philosophia Botanica* (1751) pushed this emphasis on visuality further. The book, a collection of aphorisms on botanical principles and practices, provided definitions of botanical terms as well as parameters for the naturalist's behaviour. Much of the *Philosophia* was dedicated to training the botanist as an observer and a classifier through textual and visual instruction that detailed what to look for when studying a plant. Linnaeus took a special interest in combining textual and visual instructions. The eleven plates in the book depict the different possible structural variations of each part of the plant, providing a visual botanical glossary. The first plate presented sixty-two possible leaf shapes, with the accompanying text providing a Latin term

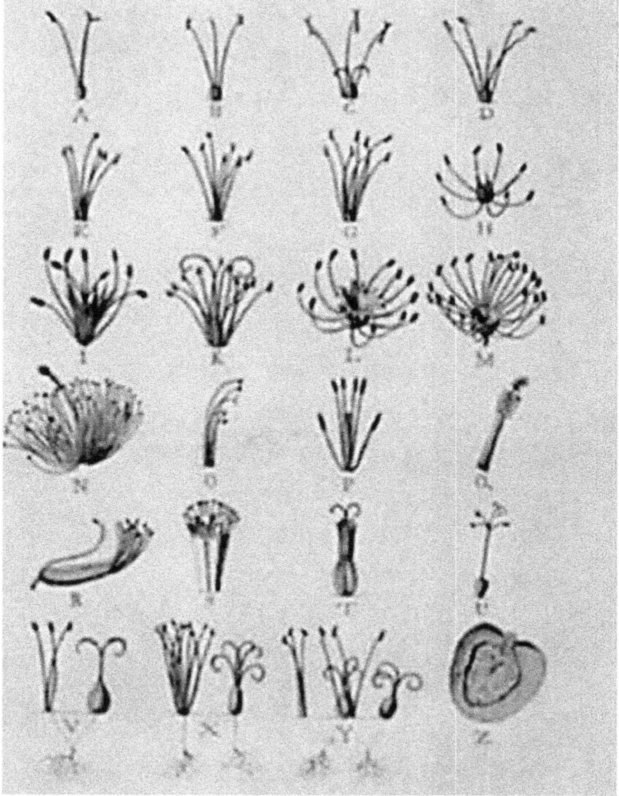

Figure 8.2 Georg Dyonisius Ehret's illustration of the twenty-four classes of the Linnaean botanical system, 1736. From Ove Hagelin, *Georg Dionysius Ehret and his Plate of the Sexual System of Plants in Linnæus' Own Copy of Systema Naturæ* (Stockholm: Hagströmer Biblioteket, The Hagströmer Medico-Historical Library, Svenska Läkaresällskapet, Karolinska Institutet, 2000). (Courtesy of the Linnean Society of London)

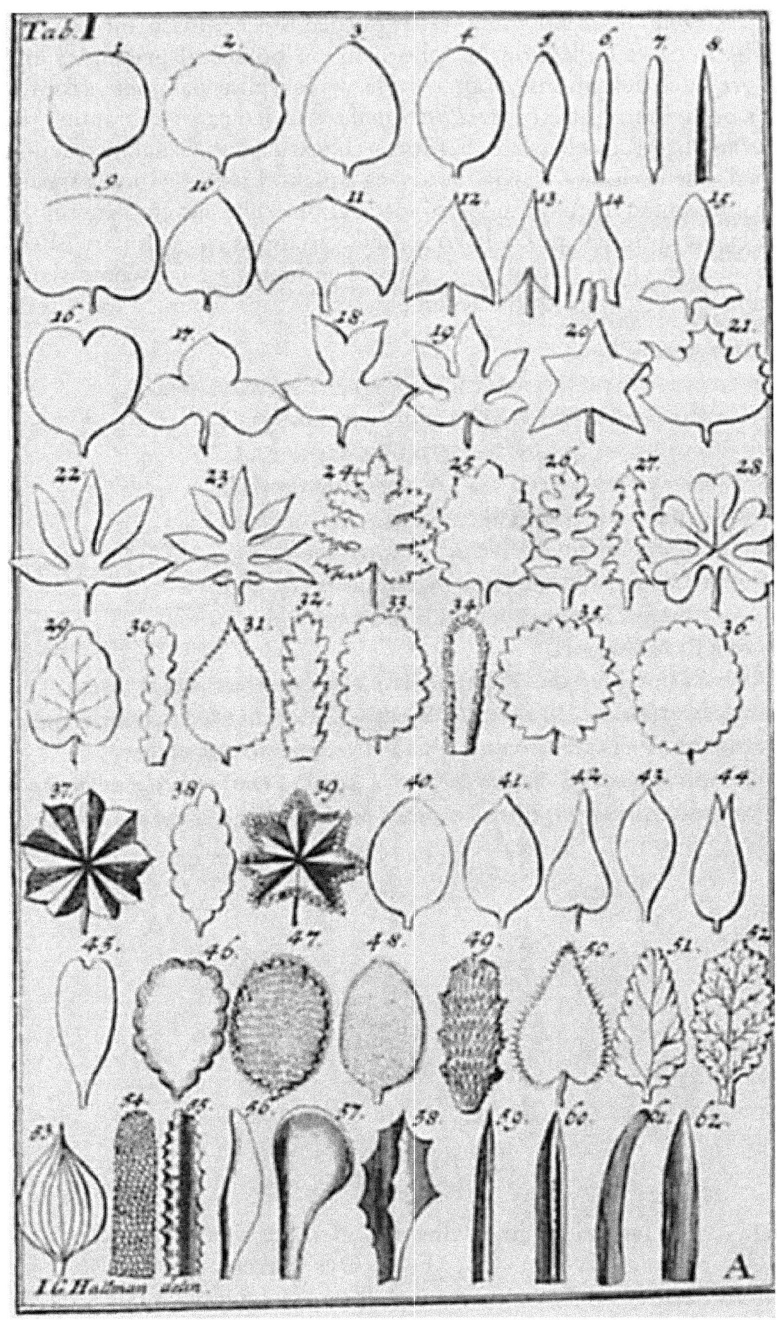

Figure 8.3 First plate of Linnaeus's *Philosophia Botanica* (Stockholm, 1751). (Courtesy of the Linnean Society of London)

for each type – specialised observation practices connected form to classification as well as to specialised terminology (Figure 8.3). The other ten plates in the book extended this visual vocabulary to offer templates for describing how the leaves are aggregated into branches, how the branch is positioned into the stem, what the roots look like, and so on, ending with a depiction of the type of wooden armoire in which herbarium specimens would be stored. These plates were copied or adapted in practically every single botanical textbook, and provided a visual and verbal vocabulary shared by naturalists throughout and beyond Europe.[9] Rather than books to read, *Systema Naturae* and *Philosophia Botanica* were books to use. Botanical eyes and botanical memories were trained through laborious exercises in viewing comparatively and establishing correspondences. Linnaeus was proposing not only a taxonomical system and a methodology based on observation, but moreover a specific type of observation, in which objects were always seen against one another. The practice of natural history involved a constant triangulation among specimens, textual information and images.

The prominence of the eye as the consummate taxonomical instrument was by no means limited to Linnaean botany but extended to other fields of natural history as well as other taxonomical approaches. Antoine-Joseph Dezallier D'Argenville's immensely popular book on conchology proposed a three-part method for classifying shells that was based on the successive visual examination of a specimen, first noting the number of parts, then establishing the overall shape of the shell, and finally identifying subtle differences in small details, patterns and colouring (1742: 123–28).[10] The volume was amply illustrated, and many of the plates served to simultaneously exemplify the identifying traits of a type of shell and to train the reader as an observer capable of noticing them. This was clearly not an easy task, given the enormous diversity within every class of shells, the minute variations that an observer needed to identify in order to distinguish among species, and the necessity to possess a visual vocabulary that could encompass every category (Figure 8.4). Likewise, the study of insects demanded specific ways of seeing and describing that would make it possible to recognise minute variations in shape, colour, and pattern and thus differentiate among insects. Thus, the image of a butterfly that opened Moses Harris's *The Aurelian* (1766) functioned as a plan specifying the different sections of a wing, which required comparative viewing in order to identify a specimen (Figure 8.5). As these illustrations make particularly clear, botanical, conchological and entomological images functioned as diagrams rather than as naturalistic portraits. They constituted idealised abstractions that eschewed the details of individual specimens to concentrate on the types of traits that an observer should be able to find and distinguish.[11]

Eighteenth-century natural history publications repeatedly insisted that vision constituted the best method for investigating nature and that images provided privileged means of transmitting this knowledge – whether through images like Rumphius's portrait, detailed instructions or direct statements

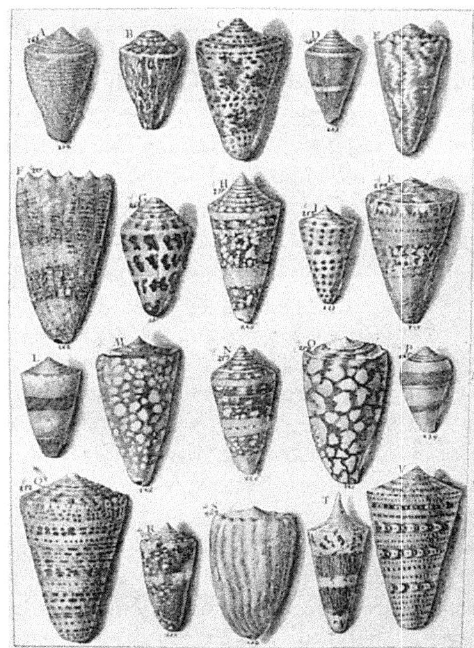

Figure 8.4 Antoine-Joseph Dezallier D'Argenville's conchology treatise, *L'Histoire naturelle, éclaircie dans deux de ses parties principales, La Lithologie et la Conchyliologie* (Paris, 1742): plate 15. (Courtesy of the Linnean Society of London)

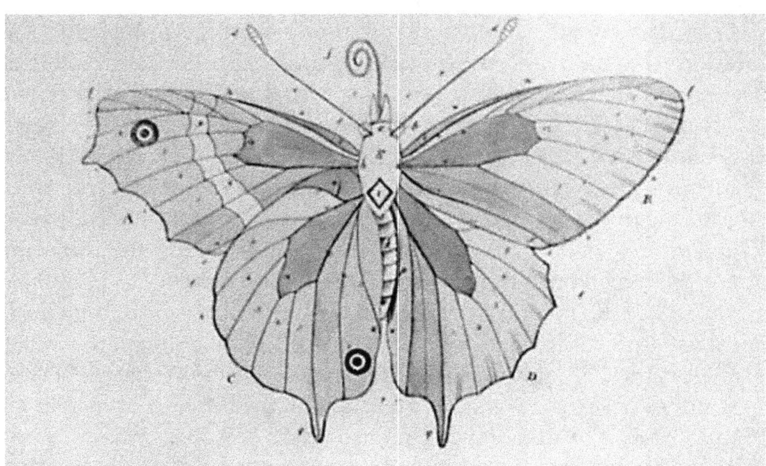

Figure 8.5 The image of a butterfly that opened Moses Harris' *The Aurelian, or Natural History of English Insects; namely Moths and Butterflies* (London, 1766), page 6. (Courtesy of the Linnean Society of London)

about the superior power of images over texts to transmit information. This was true regardless of a book's specific subject matter (botanical, entomological, conchological or other), intended audience (learned specialists or polite amateurs), language, country of publication, or any other factor – including whether the book itself contained illustrations or not, which often had more to do with publishing costs than with the perceived value of images. It is telling, after all, that one of the most successful popular natural history publications of the century was entitled *The Spectacle of Nature* (Pluché 1732-51). Buffon's *Natural History, General and Particular*, another bestseller, urged readers to 'observe, describe, and speak to the eyes, if possible by means of good figures. Those are the fundamental points that my instructions demand from you' (Latreille 1802–5, vol. 1: 52).[12] The very 'art' of the naturalist, the author explained, consisted in the capacity to observe skilfully and to render the results of an observation in a suitable manner (ibid.).[13]

The use of the term 'art,' that is of a trained and skilled set of practices involving tacit and embodied knowledge (as in the crafts), is significant.[14] Lucas Antonio Palacio's *Secretos raros de artes y oficios* ('Rare secrets of arts and trades') repeated the motif, explaining that the study of nature required great sagacity, patience and courage 'in order never to lose nature from sight, despite the great care she herself continually seems to take to hide from our view; to follow her in her progress, which is always the same under the surface but rare and infinitely varied with regards to appearances; in brief, to understand her gradual differences and the scale of her variations, which often are imperceptible to the most penetrating gaze' (Palacio 1806, vol. VI: 121).[15] The study of nature could be addressed in a publication dedicated to arts and trades, and described as a process of discovering rare secrets through a type of observation that by necessity went beyond the penetrating gaze. Something more – something else – was needed to find what lay hidden, to peek under the surface, and to understand what remained opaque even to penetrating gazes. And numerous other publications warned the observer against the treacherously deceptive first glance, which authors contrasted to the careful, reflective and comparative process of viewing that yielded true knowledge.[16] In eighteenth-century natural history, seeing was neither simple nor immediate. Viewing was a sophisticated technique that required specialised training, identified practitioners as belonging or not to a community of observers, and allowed them to evaluate the skill and talent of others. While instructions provided guidelines for observation and trained the naturalist's eye, it was a shared assumption that this eye ultimately relied more on experience and talent than on rote procedure.

Thus, working in South America in 1783, Spanish naturalist José Celestino Mutis noted in his journal that three distinct but almost identical-looking plant species could only be told apart if 'surveyed with botanical eyes' (Mutis 1983a, vol. 2: 65). In a letter from the following year, Mutis referred to Swedish naturalists Carl Linnaeus and Peter Jonas Bergius as possessing the 'delicate eyes' that characterized great botanists and made their observations trustworthy (Mutis 1983b, vol. 1: 154–56). Linnaeus himself went further in identifying the botanical eye as that elusive *je ne sais quoi* indicative of an extraordinarily talented naturalist. In a characteristically colourful aphorism, he explained: 'An experienced botanist quite often distinguishes plants from Africa, Asia, America, and the Alps, but could not easily say by what feature. I do not know what is *grim, dry, and dark* about the AFRICAN plants' appearance, what is *proud and exalted* about the ASIATIC; *what is glad and smooth* about the AMERICAN, or *compressed and hardened* about the ALPINE' (Linnaeus 2003: 131). The naturalist's gaze was not only capable of identifying all significant traits in their enormous variety and subtleness but could also function as a sort of embodied visual intuition, capturing information about the whole that could not be deduced from the sum of the parts. Given that natural investigation was construed as visual project and the naturalist identified as a specialised observer, portraits of naturalists often depicted them with images as a way of emphasising their visual expertise and skills. In such portraits, images were proudly displayed as the tools of the trade.[17]

Two final points about the naturalist's eye bear noting, even if their full discussion exceeds the purpose of this essay. The naturalist's observational skills did not reside exclusively in the eye but also in the hand. As my discussion of the use of printed illustrations suggests, viewing and representing constituted related activities. Naturalists were trained not only to observe but also to draw, and did so often and well – indeed, natural history training shared many preoccupations and methodologies with academic artistic training.[18] Dezallier D'Argenville recommended drawing shells as a way to learn to recognise and classify them. 'What better way is there to recognize all the differences among shells,' he asked, 'than to draw them from nature? The slightest fold, the subtleties in the shape of a contour, of the mouth: nothing can escape, and nothing can better reveal the shell's true character' (1742: 117). Thus, drawing promised a solution to the problem of capturing the ever-elusive mysteries of nature.

Furthermore, the comparative eyes of the taxonomist found their counterpart in the appraising eyes of the connoisseur. Like naturalists, collectors were expert observers trained to identify objects accurately, distinguishing among very similar ones based on minuscule differences. Dutch apothecary Albertus Seba, to name but one noted eighteenth-century collector, owned a remarkable collection of natural history specimens and images. He had them engraved and published as *Locupletissimi Rerum Naturalium Thesauri* (1734–65). The portrait included in the work (Figure 8.6) shows Seba holding in his right hand a glass jar with a specimen preserved in spirits, and pointing with his left hand to shell and mineral specimens that lie on the table next to an open book with drawings of insects and animals. Seba's gaze, unremittingly fixed on the viewer, forms the third point of a triangle: the eyes that observe, the hand that shows and the hand that owns.

The positioning of the body to one side of the image with the arms stretched out towards the opposite side, and the placement of the hands add an implicit directionality to these three points, travelling from the eyes to the pointing hand to the holding hand, in this way recreating the trajectory of objects through observation, collection and possession. Seba's placement between the objects and images slightly before him and the collection of jars behind him reinforces this depiction of him as intermediary: with one hand he can reach forth to gather natural objects, with the other, he can reach back to place them within the ordered shelves of European science.

Seba's portrait also reminds us of the importance of the collection, or the cabinet, as a repository not only of natural history in its various material incarnations – as specimens, books, images – but also of colonial and imperial experiences. Many of the natural productions depicted in illustrations or displayed in cabinets were the result of colonial ventures. In the remainder of this chapter, I would like to suggest some connections between the visual culture of nature and its colonial exploitation.

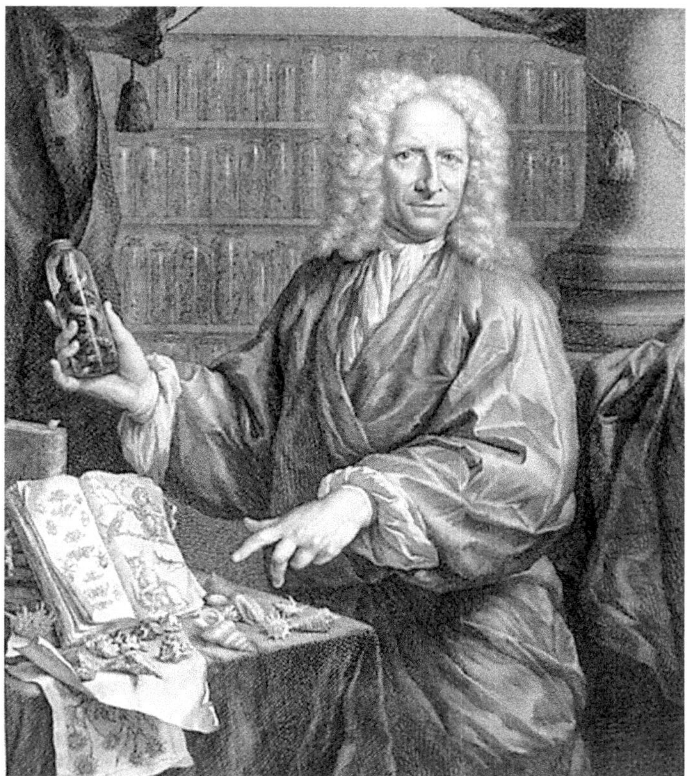

Figure 8.6 Portrait of Albertus Seba. Frontmatter of his *Locupletissimi rerum naturalium thesauri* (Amsterdam, 1734-65), vol. 1. (Courtesy of the Linnean Society of London)

Contrasting Views: Global White Space, Local Colour

Opening the cover of Rumphius's *Amboinese Curiosity Cabinet* (1705), the reader encounters an impressively engraved frontispiece (Figure 8.7). Within a splendid neoclassical setting, a scene unfolds in three spatial acts. In the foreground, servants have gathered a rich collection of natural specimens, among them a giant crab and many large shells. A semi-naked servant carries a basket and a box with specimens into the middle ground, where scholars gather around a table deep in discussion as they examine objects that have been brought to them, using books to assist their observations. To either side of the table, large cabinets attest to the magnitude of this project of accumulation. In the background, assistants store the collected objects in the drawers of yet another large cabinet. Through the open windows of this last room, we are able to glimpse the outside world from where these specimens were plucked. The engraving represents the processes involved in the study of

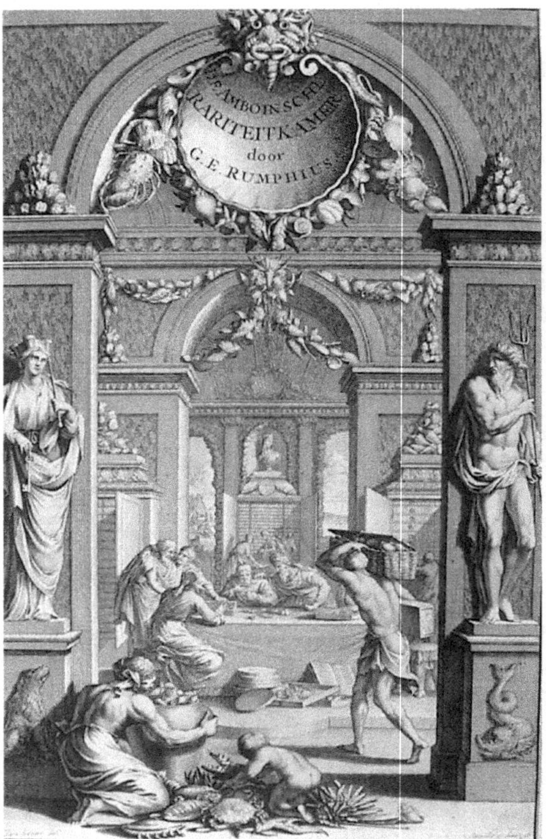

Figure 8.7 Engraved frontispiece of Rumphius's *Amboinese curiosity cabinet* (Amsterdam, 1705). (Courtesy of the Linnean Society of London)

nature –collection, observation and classification. It also traces the trajectories of objects as they penetrate the sphere of European science. What is remarkably absent from this idealised depiction of the study of nature is any kind of lack of activity taking place outside, in the field. We encounter natural products already plucked and transported indoors. Though Rumphius spent most of his adult life in the Dutch East Indies, this colonial setting is erased from his book's frontispiece and from his portrait, both of which are interior scenes. Colonial nature is literally out of the picture.

This is also the case with the illustrations within the book, which accompanied textual descriptions of the natural products Rumphius collected in Ambon (Figure 8.8). Regardless of the objects represented, images showed decontextualised, isolated specimens upon the white background of the page. These illustrations did not depict living organisms but collectible specimens. This pictorial convention privileged the material integrity and specificity of the natural specimen, understood as an object whose value resided in its appearance and its relationship to other natural objects in an aesthetic arrangement. The vast majority of illustrations portrayed specimens in

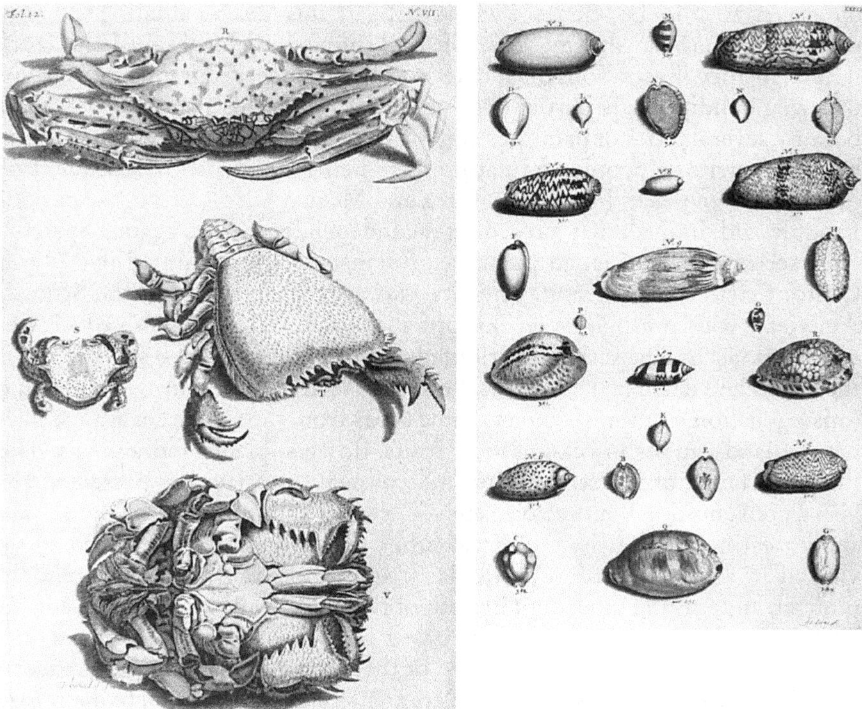

Figure 8.8 Rumphius, Georg Everhard, *De Amboinsche rariteitkamer* (Amsterdam, 1705): Plates 7 and 39. (Courtesy of the Linnean Society of London)

standard views and positions, placed on the white page almost as if they were objects in a cabinet drawer. More than depicted, creatures were displayed. And, while the distant and exotic provenance of the items made them more rare, thus adding to their price and value, this was impossible to deduce from the image itself.

Such decontextualisation was the norm for seventeenth- and eighteenth-century natural history illustrations. For the most part, these images consisted of a few ink traces floating on a sea of white, the overwhelmingly blank page. Given the impressive powers of the naturalist's eyes to identify and classify, to see the invisible (as Linnaeus suggested), or even to see without seeing (as in the case of Rumphius), it is remarkable just how much these trained eyes chose not to see and not to show. Observation and representation operated within the parameters of other natural history practices of the time, such as reading, collecting and classifying, all of which were based on methods of comparison, evaluation, criticism and, importantly, selection. The naturalist's gaze was extraordinarily selective not only about what it noticed but also about what it disregarded.

This selectivity, I argue, represented an exclusionary strategy intimately connected to colonial science. I will investigate this idea by alluding to a case study from the Spanish Americas. The exclusion of any local specificity from natural history illustrations, be it in terms of landscape, geography, or cultural or social conditions, is particularly noteworthy for this region at that time because several types of paintings emphasising precisely the interconnections between territory, people and nature were being developed independent of one another in places like Quito, Lima and Mexico City – this is the period, I should add, immediately preceding the independence wars against Spain.[19]

A series of six unsigned paintings, for instance, was painted in 1783 in Quito, Ecuador (figure 8.9). The city was an artistic centre in the Spanish Americas, with prestigious workshops that produced highly valued secular and religious art The series is attributed to Vicente Albán, who signed one of the works and dated it. The images, known collectively as *cuadros de mestizaje* (miscegenation paintings), depict ethnic types from the region set against lush natural landscapes showcasing local fruits, flowers, plants and animals. The flora and fauna of the region, ripe and colourful, are lavishly presented for visual consumption – more concretely, in two of the paintings the figures are shown eating fruit. It is unclear whether the images were designed to be viewed in a specific order, particularly since only two of them include a number, and it is the same digit in both of them. However, the series seems to break into three pairs of paintings based on the social types depicted, the positioning of the figures (and, in two of the three instances, of the cartouche as well), and the text describing the contents of each picture. The paintings relate the region's inhabitants to its flora and fauna, and also construct an idealised social order by contrasting opposed human pairs between and within the images. Thus, the painting depicting an *Yndio principal* in lavish dress in the foreground also includes a small figure in the background labelled *Yndio del campo*, or field Indian. This is also the case with the *Yndia en trage de gala* (Indian woman dressed up in finery), who is contrasted against a female field Indian, or the *Señora principal* depicted with her black slave. After such displays of finery, the final two paintings of the series push the juxtapositions even further by presenting two barely dressed Amerindian men.

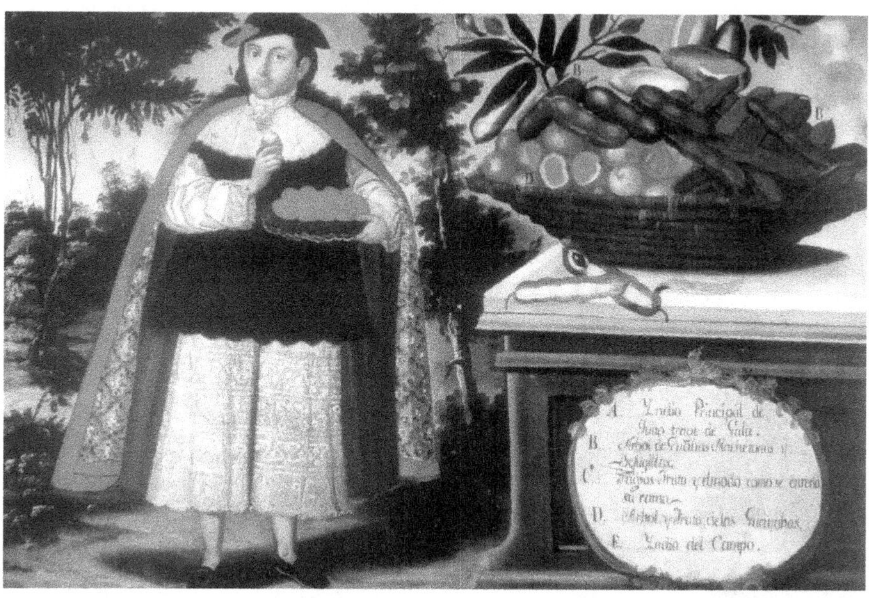

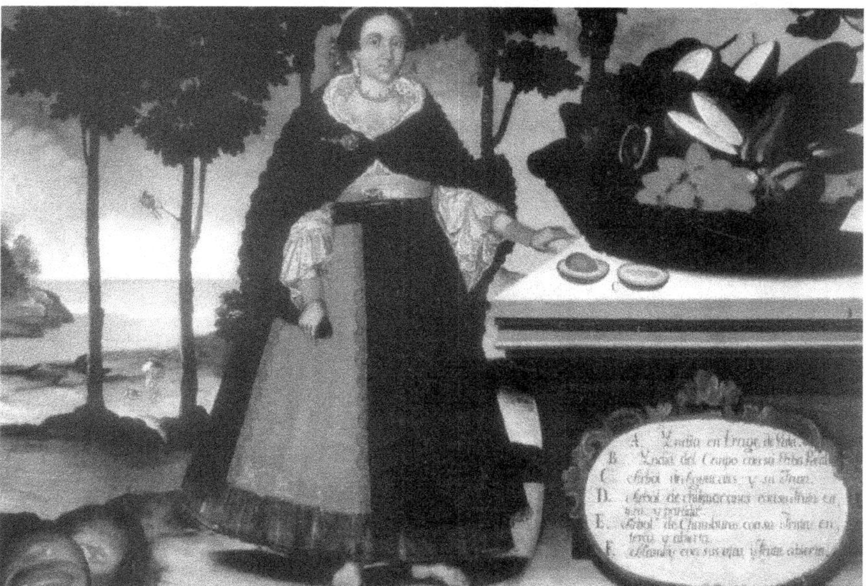

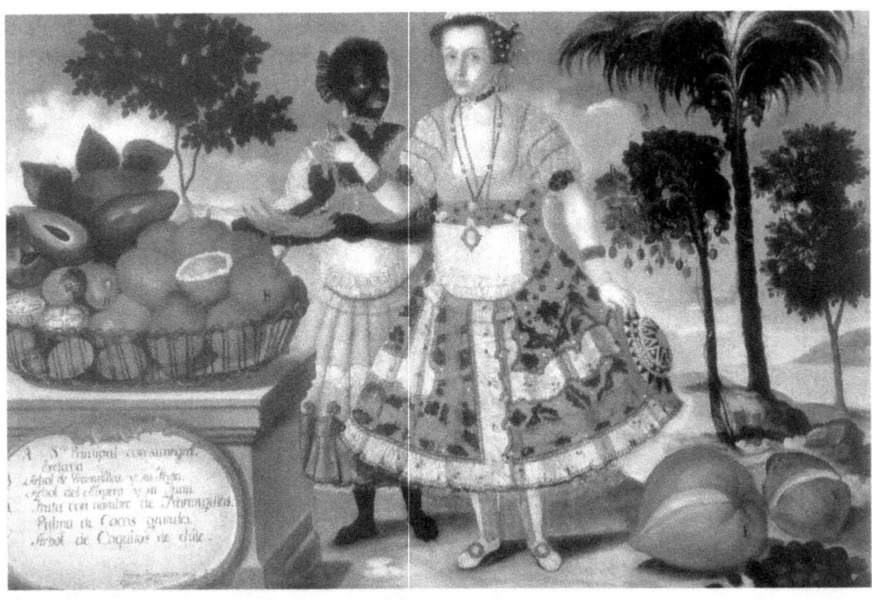

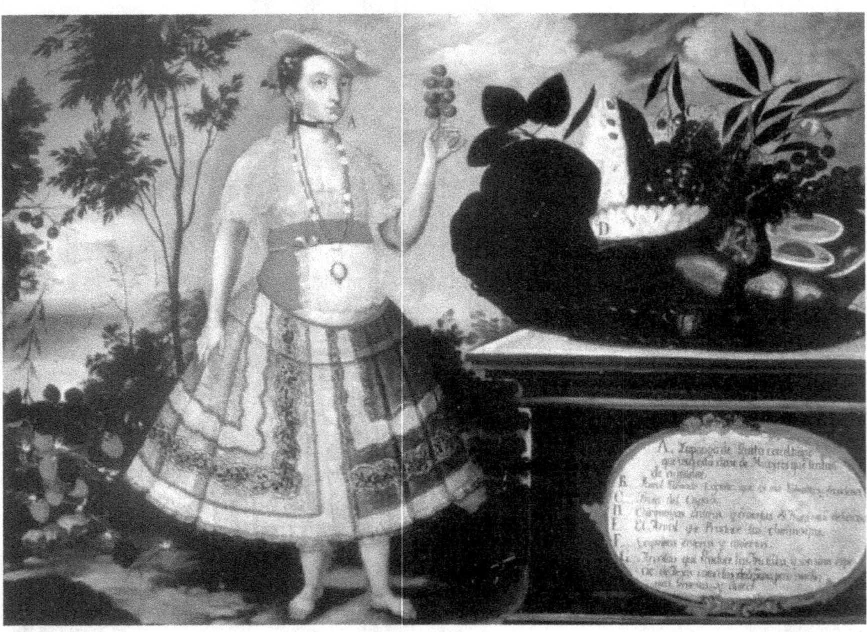

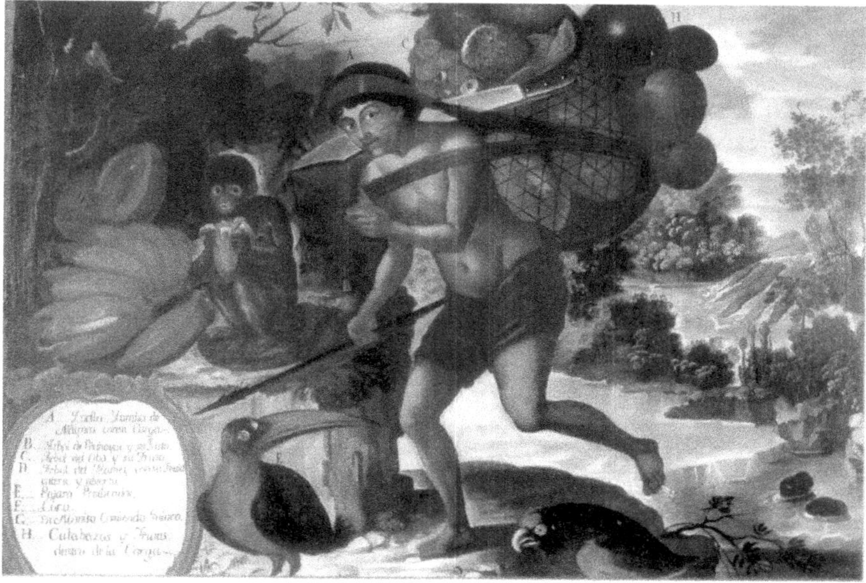

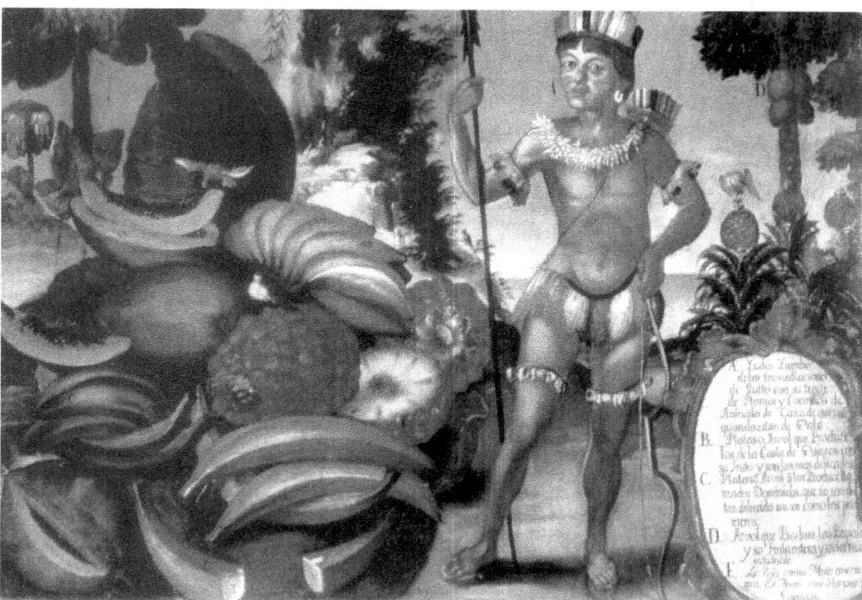

Figure 8.9 Vicente Albán, *Cuadros de mestizaje* (Quito, 1783). (Courtesy of the Museo de América, Madrid)

The most famous series of human types in Spanish-American colonial painting are the *casta* paintings developed in Mexico in the eighteenth century.[20] Produced in most cases in series of sixteen images, these paintings present combinations of couples of different ethnicities with an offspring. Settings can be domestic or exterior, urban or rural, but a significant proportion include flora and fauna. The number sixteen is significant, since it alludes to the four generations that needed to be taken into account in order to calculate a person's *calidad* (quality) according to their *limpieza de sangre* (blood purity or cleanliness). A written inscription in each panel indicated the parents' ethnicity and provided the appropriate label for the child coming from that mix. Thus, *casta* paintings presented an ethnic hierarchy that privileged white over indigenous over black, and correlated this gradation to wealth, occupation, social standing, and even happiness – in some series, the darkest-hued families are engaged in alarming acts of domestic violence. *Casta* paintings ordered nature and society into an idealised taxonomy.[21] These images addressed one of the great fears of colonial societies in the Spanish Americas by suggesting that ethnicity was not fluid and easily confused but rather mathematically fixed, compartmentalised and readily identifiable visually. Given that *casta* paintings portrayed highly local categories of social order, and presented them as arising from a natural order, the fact that people were accompanied by local natural productions is highly relevant.

The connections among human populations, social order, natural productions and territory are clearly demonstrated in an oil painting entitled *A Painting of the Natural, Civil, and Geographical History of the Kingdom of Peru* (Figure 8.10, Barras de Aragón 1912). An artist named Luis Thiebaut painted it in Peru in 1799, most probably commissioned by José Ignacio Lequanda, who signed the 'preliminary address' included in the work and dedicated it to the Spanish *Real Hacienda de Indias*. This very large painting (325 × 115 cm) offers a visual microcosm of the colony. Eighty-eight cells with images of birds and plants provide an outer frame to the composition,

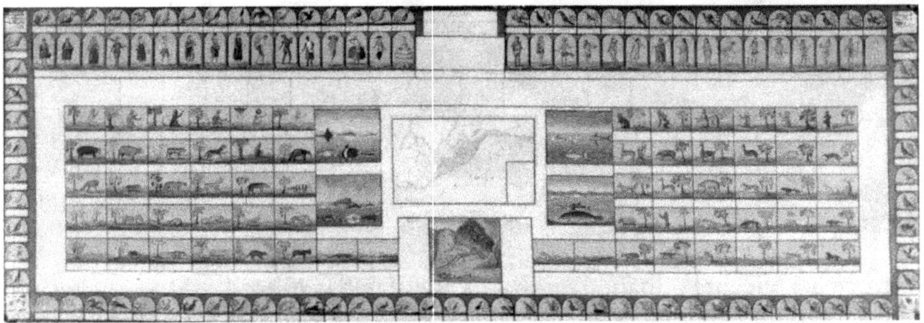

Figure 8.10 Luis Thiebaut, 1799, *A Painting of the Natural, Civil, and Geographical History of the Kingdom of Peru.* (Courtesy of the Museo Nacional de Ciencias Naturales, Madrid)

with the four corners dedicated to insects. An internal textual belt examines the history of Peru from the Inca empire to the present, pointing out notable events and describing each region of the kingdom as well as the temperament of its inhabitants. Immediately above it appear thirty-two human types. The sixteen cells on the left depict 'civilised nations', while the sixteen on the right show 'savage nations'. Most human figures are presented in male–female pairs. The entire ethnic and social gradation of colonial society is depicted: the 'civilised nations' include different indigenous groups, African and American blacks, mulattos – described for the intended peninsular viewer as the American equivalent to European gypsies – and the *criollos de Lima,* that is, Peruvian-born descendants of Europeans. The various indigenous groups depicted as 'savage nations' are presented as noble savages. They might not have adopted Christianity, but they are not the barbaric carnivores common in sixteenth-century images. Rather, they are shown with babies, fishing or hunting instruments, or local animals. Significantly, Europeans are not included in the painting. The centre of the painting is occupied by a geographical map of Peru and a view of the mine of Gualgayoc or Chota. To either side of the map and mine are two cells with aquatic creatures and thirty cells with animals and plants. All these cells show local plants and animals, describing in Spanish their local names, regions where they grow, and uses. This unusual work combines text with images from different pictorial genres.[22] Like the taxonomical publication or the natural history cabinet, it aims for order and completion. The great difference is that while European scientific images and collections dissociate natural objects from the territories they came from, this painting situates and integrates. The natural, civil and geographical history of the kingdom complement one another. Flora and fauna are presented in conjunction, united in the same image. The pictures of people attempt to provide a total view of Peru's inhabitants, presenting them as separate but connected.

European natural history illustrations present a paradox as great as that of the blind observer. The very point of the publications in which they appeared was to place before European eyes little-known natural products from distant lands. Specimens were collected, described, drawn and published precisely because they grew in Asia, North America and South America. The actual place of origin, however, never appeared in their depictions – although textual descriptions did note it. The visual omission is significant, and reminds us that eighteenth-century natural history not only insisted on the centrality of vision but also demanded that views always remain partial. More than mere representations, images acted as visual avatars replacing perishable or untransportable objects that would otherwise remain unseen and unknown by Europeans. Working in South America for over forty years, Spanish naturalist José Celestino Mutis articulated the potential of images to allow long-distance knowing-by-seeing in a letter in which he explained that 'no plant, from the loftiest tree to the humblest weed, will remain hidden to the investigation of true botanists if represented after nature for the instruction of those who, unable to travel throughout the world, without seeing plants in their native soil will be able to know them through their detailed explanation and living image' (Mutis 1983b, vol. 1: 316).[23] Images preserved the impermanent and transported the distant. More than illustrations or representations, they came to stand in for the objects they depicted, providing European naturalists with visual repertoires that allowed them to gather and compare natural specimens from around the world within the enclosed spaces of their studies.

In this way, natural history illustrations defined nature as a series of transportable objects whose identity and importance was divorced from the environment where they grew or the culture of its inhabitants. Pictures were used to reject the local as contingent, subjective and translatable, favouring instead the dislocated global as objective, truthful and permanent. The Linnaean system proposed a totalising, universal way of seeing as well as of classifying. And it did so quite self-consciously: in his *Critica Botanica*, Linnaeus wrote: 'Native locality does not make a specific difference. Locality neither canonizes nor changes anyone; as the proverb goes, not even a pig is changed by being taken to Rome' (1737: 130). Faced with a multitude of overlapping taxonomies and nomenclatures, naturalists were relieved to have a single system, a single naming method, and a single visual approach that remained operative regardless of where it was employed or by whom. Images showed decontextualised specimens, uprooted from their native soils, expunged from any use or cultural context. The ordered list of Latin names and descriptions and the illustration of isolated specimens on blank pages served to cleanse the soil out of nature, transforming local productions into delocalised natural specimens.

Notes

1 On the importance of print to early modern science, see Frasca-Spada and Jardine (2000).

2 Paula Findlen describes a similar role for books in sixteenth-century natural history (1999).

3 Daston and Park examine the transformation in attitudes towards nature and its investigation from the mid-twelfth century to the mid-eighteenth century (1998), with a particular concern for changes in epistemology. On the connections among collecting, display and natural history in early modern Europe, see Findlen (1994) and Bredekamp (1995).

4 'Si nous examinons attentivement ce peuple nouveau & entierement oublié [coquillages], si nous considérons en particulier chacun des êtres qui le composent, nous découvrirons dans leurs moeurs, dans leurs actions, dans leurs mouvements, dans leur manière de vivre, une infinité de choses très-curieuses, des faits intéressants & capables de fixer l'attention d'un observateur avide & intelligent.'

5 'J'admire le courage de ces voyageurs qui, pour accroître nos collections, bravent les fureurs du vaste Océan, et récoltent à travers mille dangers … des animaux et des plantes rares ou inconnues; mais je pense que la zoologie gagneroit davantage, si d'habiles observateurs, se répandant dans différentes parties du monde, en étudioient, à demeure et pendant plusieurs années, les richesses naturelles.'

6 Justin Stagl discusses a comparable (and related) concern with the methodical training of the traveller's skills as an observer and a describer over the early-modern period (1995). For

instance, Nathan Chytraeus summarised his instructions on travel methodology (*Variorum in Europa Itinerum Deliciae*, 1594) in the form of a chart (reproduced in Stagl 1995: 61).

7 Ehret's original drawings for the plate are held at the Natural History Museum, London. The printed plate of 1736 is known to exist in only three copies, including Linnaeus' own copy of the first edition of the *Systema Naturae* (1735), held at the Hagströmer Medico-Historical Library of the Swedish Society of Medicine, in the Karolinska Institutet, Stockholm, Sweden (Hagelin 2000). On Ehret, who produced the engravings for some of the century's most celebrated travel accounts and natural histories, see Blunt (1951, chap. 12); Bray (1989: 62–85, 107–19); Calmann (1977); and Ehret (1987).

8 On Linnaean classification, see Blunt (2001), Koerner (1999), Larson (1994) and Stafleu (1971). On gender and the Linnaean sexual system of classification, see Schiebinger (1993, 1996).

9 Among many other works, versions of these plates appear in Philip Millers, *Garderner's Dictionary* (1st edn. 1724, 8th edn. 1768); Antoine Gouan, *Hortus Regius Monspeliensis* (Leiden, 1762); John Millers, *An Illustration of the Sexual System of Linnaeus*, 2 vols (London, 1779); Casimiro Gómez Ortega and Antonio Palaus, *Curso elemental de botánica, teórico y práctico, dispuesto para la enseñanza del Real Jardín Botánico* (Madrid, 1785, 2nd rev. edn. 1795).

10 On conchological illustration, including D'Argenville's, see Spary (2004).

11 The implications posed in the choice between illustrating one particular specimen and providing a composite image that represented an idealised type is discussed by Daston and Galison (1992).

12 'Observez, décrivez et parlez aux yeux, s'il est possible, par le moyen de bonnes figures; tels sont les points fondamentaux sur lesquels vous réclamex mes instructions.'

13 'Bien observer, et rendre d'une manière couvenable ce qu'on a vu, c'est en cela que consiste tout l'art du naturaliste.'

14 The close relationship between art, artisanal practices and early modern science is ellaborated in Smith (2004).

15 'Para estudiar bien la naturaleza, se necesita mucha sagacidad, paciencia y aun valor: sagacidad para no perder nunca de vista la naturaleza, á pesar de los cuidados que parece que ella misma toma para esconderse continuamente à nuestra vista; para seguirla en su progreso, siempre igual en el fondo, pero rara y variada á lo infinito en quanto á las apariencias, en fin, para comprehender sus diferencias graduales, y la escala de sus variedades, muchas veces imperceptibles á la vista más penetrante.' I am grateful to Nuria Valverde for sharing this quote with me.

16 These concerns were shared by collectors of naturalia. In his catalogue to Pedro Franco Dávila's natural history collection, Jean-Baptiste-Louis Romé de L'Isle explained that although at first glance ('au premier coup d'oeil') shell fossils might appear identical to contemporary organisms, a careful comparison would almost always make differences evident (1767, vol. II: 49).

17 There seem to be prevalent two iconographies of the naturalist in the late eighteenth century, showing him (for the naturalist is almost invariably a he) discretely holding a flower or branch of a plant named in his honour, or pointing to an illustration of a plant. Given that the first convention was also commonly employed in portraits of gentlemen and women, where plants or flowers were included among several other visual symbols alluding to the sitter's refinement, sophistication or character, I interpret the choice to depict naturalists not with actual plants but with their illustrations as an appeal to their status as specialised practitioners, akin to the representation of astronomers or cosmographers with scientific instruments. On scientific portraiture, see Jordanova (2000).

18 On art training see Goldstein (1996) and Boschloo *et al.* (1989).

19 On the connections between Creole identity, nationalism, science and the independence wars, see Brading (1991), Cañizares-Esguerra (2001) and Glick (1991).

20 On *casta* paintings, see Katzew (1996, 2004) and Carrera (2003).

21 On eighteenth-century racial thinking, see Hudson (1996) and Vyverberg (1989).

22 There exist at least two other South American iconographic collections that present local views of nature, which I hope to analyse in future work. One is a group of eighty-six zoological images commissioned by Lázaro de Ribera, governor of the region of Moxos in Peru, and sent to Madrid between 1786 and 1794 to accompany his reports to the crown (Ribera 1989). The other is a collection of watercolours commissioned by Baltasar Jaime Martínez Compañón, bishop of the diocesis of Trujillo, Peru, who travelled through the viceroyalty between 1779 and 1789 accompanied by cartographers and artists. The 1,411 drawings illuminated in watercolour were gathered in nine volumes, six of which are dedicated to natural history (Martínez Compañón 1978–94; López Serrano 1976).

23 'Por este medio se va logrando que no quede oculta a la investigación de los verdaderos botánicos planta desde el árbol más elevado hasta la yerba más humilde, y representada al natural para la instrucción de los que no puediendo viajar por todo el mundo, sin ver las plantas en su suelo nativo podrán conocerlas por circunstanciada explicación y viva imagen.'

References

Primary sources

Adanson, M. 1757. *Histoire naturelle du Sénégal. Coquillages. Avec la Relation abrégée d'un Voyage fait en ce pays, pendant les années 1749, 50, 51, 52 & 53.* Paris.

Aublet, F. 1775. *Histoire des plantes de la Guiane Françoise.* London.

Dezallier D'Argenville, A.-J. 1742. *L'Histoire naturelle, éclaircie dans deux de ses parties principales, La Lithologie et la Conchyliologie.* Paris.

Ehret, G.D. 1987. *Ehret's Flowering Plants.* London.

Latreille, P.A. 1802–1805. *Histoire naturelle, générale et particuliere des crustacés et des insectes. Ouvrage faisant suite aux Oeuvres de Leclerc de Buffon.* Paris.

Linnaeus, C. 1737. *Critica Botanica.* Leiden.

———. 2003. *Philosophia Botanica* [1751], trans. Stephen Freer. Oxford.

Moses, H. 1766. *The Aurelian, or Natural History of English Insects; namely Moths and Butterflies.* London.

Mutis, J.C. 1983a. *Diario de observaciones de José Celestino Mutis (1760–1790),* transcription and prol. by Guillermo Hernández de Alba, 2nd edn. Bogota.

———. 1983b. *Archivo epistolar del sabio naturalista Don José C. Mutis,* ed. Guillermo Hernández de Alba. 2nd edn. Bogota.

Palacio, L.A. de. 1806. *Secretos raros de artes y oficios. Obra útil a toda clase de personas.* 3rd edn. Madrid.

Pluché, N.-A. 1732–51. *Le spectacle de la nature*. Paris.

Ribera, L. de. 1989. *Moxos: descripciones exactas e historia fiel de los indios, animales y plantas de la provincia de Moxos en el Virreinato del Perú por Lázaro de Ribera, 1786-1794.* Facs. edn. Madrid.

Romé de L'Isle, J.-B.-L. 1767. *Catalogue systématique et raisonné des curiosités de la nature et de l'art, qui composent le cabinet de M. Davila, avec figures en taille douce.* Paris.

Rumphius, G.E. 1999. *The Ambonese Curiosity Cabinet* [*De Amboinsche rariteitkamer*, 1705], trans., ed., anno. and with an intro. by E.M. Beekman. New Haven and London.

———. 1741–50. *Herbarium Amboinense,* ed. Johann Burmann. Amsterdam.

———. 1755. *Herbarii Amboinensis Auctuarium.* Amsterdam.

Seba, A. 1734–65. *Locupletissimi Rerum Naturalium Thesauri.* Amsterdam.

Secondary sources

Barras de Aragón, F. de las. 1912. 'Una historia del Perú contenida en un cuadro al óleo de 1799'. *Boletín de la Real Sociedad Española de Historia Natural*, XII: 224–85. Madrid.

Blunt, W. 1951. *The Art of Botanical Illustration.* London.

——. 2001. *The Compleat Naturalist. A Life of Linnaeus*, intro. William T. Stearn. 2nd edn. London.

Boschloo, Anton, *et al.*, eds. 1989. *Academies of Art. Between Renaissance and Romanticism.* The Hague.

Brading, D. 1991. *The First America: the Spanish Monarchy, Creole Patriots, and the Liberal State, 1492–1867.* Cambridge, UK.

Bray, L. de. 1989. *The Art of Botanical Illustration. The Classic Illustrators and their Achievements from 1550 to 1900.* London.

Bredekamp, H. 1995. *The Lure of Antiquity and the Cult of the Machine: The Kunstkammer and the Evolution of Nature, Art and Technology*, trans. A. Brown. Princeton, NJ.

Calmann, G. 1977. *Ehret, Flower Painter Extraordinary. An Illustrated Biography.* Boston.

Cañizares-Esguerra, J. 2001. *How to Write the History of the New World: Histories, Epistemologies, and Identities in the Eighteenth-century Atlantic World.* Stanford.

Carrera, M. 2003. *Imagining Identity in New Spain: Race, Lineage, and the Colonial Body in Portraiture and Casta Paintings.* Austin.

Daston, L. and P. Galison, 1992. 'The Image of Objectivity'. *Representations* 40: 81–128.

Daston, L. and K. Park. 1998. *Wonders and the Order of Nature, 1150–1750.* New York.

Findlen, P. 1994. *Possessing Nature: Museums, Collecting, and Scientific Culture in Early Modern Italy.* Berkeley.

——. 1999. 'The Formation of a Scientific Community: Natural History in Sixteenth-century Italy', in *Natural Particulars. Nature and the Disciplines in Renaissance Europe*, eds. A. Grafton and N. Siraisi. Cambridge, Mass., 369–400.

Frasca-Spada, M. and N. Jardine, eds. 2000. *Books and the Sciences in History.* Cambridge.

Glick, T. 1991. 'Science and Independence in Latin America (with Special Reference to New Granada)'. *Hispanic American Historical Review*, 71: 307–34.

Goldstein, C. 1996. *Teaching Art. Academies and Schools from Vasari to Albers.* New York.

Hagelin, O. 2000. *Georg Dionysius Ehret and His Plate of the Sexual System of Plants in Linnaeus' Own Copy of Systema Naturae.* Stockholm.

Hudson, N. 1996. 'From "Nation" to "Race": The Origin of Racial Classification in Eighteenth-Century Thought', *Eighteenth-Century Studies*, 29: 247–64.

Jordanova, L. 2000. *Defining Features: Scientific and Medical Portraits.* London.

Katzew, I. 1996. *New World Orders: Casta Painting and Colonial Latin America.* New York.

——. 2004. *Casta Painting. Images of Race in Eighteenth-Century Mexico.* New Haven, Conn.

Koerner, L. 1999. *Linnaeus. Nature and Nation.* Cambridge, Mass.

Larson, J.L. 1994. *Interpreting Nature: the Science of Living Form from Linnaeus to Kant.* Baltimore.

Schiebinger, L. 1993. *Nature's Body: Gender in the Making of Modern Science.* Boston.

———. 1996. 'Gender and Natural History', in *Cultures of Natural History*, eds. N. Jardine, J.A. Secord and E.C. Spary. Cambridge, UK, 163–77.

Smith, P.H. 2004. *The Body of the Artisan: Art and Experience in the Scientific Revolution.* Chicago.

Spary, E.C. 2004. 'Scientific Symmetries', *History of Science*, xlii, pt. 1, no. 135: 1–46.

Stafleu, F.A. 1971. *Linnaeus and the Linneans: the Spreading of Their Ideas in Systematic Botany, 1735–1789.* Utrecht.

Stagl, J. 1995. *A History of Curiosity. The Theory of Travel, 1550–1800.* Chur.

Vyverberg, H. 1989. *Human Nature, Cultural Diversity, and the French Enlightenment.* Oxford.

Chapter 9

Navigating the Brainscape: When Knowing Becomes Seeing

Andreas Roepstorff

Introduction

Images of brains with colourful areas lighting up are a well-known outcome of functional brain scans. These images serve several concurrent purposes. They are an integral part of the research process, since they allow for the representation of very large datasets in a visual illustration that may be explored dynamically. They are important signs of evidence for those scientific papers, which are the rationale of the research. Finally, they are also aesthetic objects, carefully tailored to look 'nice' both to the scientific insider and the scientific outsider. In none of these instances can the images be considered realistic photographs. Rather, they are to be seen as ideograms – or *Sinnbilder* in Ludwik Fleck's sense – that is, as particular carriers of meaning. But how do these images come to carry meaning in the first place? In this chapter, I will examine how, during the analysis of an experiment, the 'raw images' become embedded in a narrative. From the point of view of a junior researcher, this is a process of learning how to 'read' images. That is, it is an education of attention which through directed perception allows one to 'see' the image as part of a larger narrative. This is a social process – not only because the training takes place in a social environment, but more importantly because that narrative, which the pictures are going to be embedded in, need to take into account other narratives, which the picture could evoke in the imagined community of peers. This suggests that the education of attention, which allows for skilled vision, is a key process in establishing the borders of the scientific community.

Seeing as Knowing

In the summer of 1998, I experienced what seemed to me a prototypical instance of 'enskilment of vision'. I was at fieldwork in west-central Greenland in the northern part of the Disko Bay together with a fishery biologist (Roepstorff 2003). We were travelling in a small 14' dinghy powered by an outboard motor in the Torssukkattak Icefjord. As the name suggests, there was a lot of ice around; floating out from the glaciers in the bottom of the fjord. The boat was navigated by two of our local collaborators, a fisherman and his fifteen-year-old son. They came from a nearby village, and the father had long ago decided that this, his oldest son, was the one who had the greatest inclination and skills to take on the fishery. Navigating through ice-filled waters is never easy, and even less so when you are literally standing with your feet below the level of the sea, in the bottom of a small dinghy. The icescape changes constantly as smaller and larger floes move among each other.

The biologist and I could do nothing but look out and enjoy the wonderful scenery, while the father and the son concentrated on getting us through the ever-changing labyrinth, the son by the steering handle of the motor, the father standing beside him. None of us had much to say, but every now and then, the father would nod in one direction or another, as if pointing out something. Sometimes the son nodded as well, sometimes not, but it was as if he took whatever was there into account in his planning our way through the waters.

It seems almost too straightforward to analyse this process as an enskilment through 'education of attention' (Gibson 1979; see discussion in Ingold 2001, 2003). The experienced father does not tell his son what to do, but indexically, he points out that there is something to pay attention to. This allows the son to focus in on a smaller part of that vast icescape in front of him and take whatever measures necessary. At times, the nodding seemed to point to a possible route between the floes, at others to point to something to look out for, perhaps the apparent passage was about to close or there was a potentially dangerous iceberg. We were never told, neither was the son; very few direct messages were exchanged, but through the ongoing sharing of attention, we got safely through the ice-filled waters. At the same time, the son learned something about how to see for himself, and how to act accordingly (see also Pálsson 1994, 2000).

It is a long way from Torssukkattak Icefjord to the brain scans in the title of this chapter. I chose to begin in this almost archetypal anthropological setting – in a boat with some natives in a remote part of the world – because there seem to be parallel mechanisms at play in the two instances: mechanisms that may be easier to identify in the remote setting than in the laboratory next door. In this chapter I will argue that seeing is not just seeing since identification of particular patterns requires skill, and these skills have to be learned. This appears to be the case both in the laboratory and on the icefjord. However, I would also like to bring out some differences between these two settings for skilled vision. In one instance nature is there, as it is, and the knowledge required to deal with it is there; learning to see therefore becomes a matter of learning to pay attention to some differences while down-playing others. In a simplified sense, seeing *is* knowing: once you see, you know, as indicated by the silent pointing of the father.

In the other instance, the image itself is constructed in particular ways, and the purpose of the image is to become embedded in a narrative, an article, to be circulated among peers who should, hopefully, come to agree on the knowledge which the picture is taken to represent. Perhaps somewhat paradoxically, both the seeing and the knowing in the laboratory thereby come to appear even more socially constructed than in the icefjord, and, as I will try to argue in the following, knowing becomes a prerequisite for seeing.

The Symbolicity of Brain Scans

We recently held a master-class in the brain imaging laboratory that I work in. The master was a well-known neuropsychologist, who was invited to comment on some of our research. However, in these days of fluid hierarchies, a putative master should ideally prove himself as such. We therefore decided to put him to a test: based on a series of images which depicted the outcome of a brain imaging experiment, he should pass a test on 'reverse engineering', that is, he should try to identify the experiment that could have produced these images. This is not easy, and in order for you to follow what it takes, I will very briefly present a crash course in brain imaging (see Frackowiak 2004 for a thorough overview of concepts and methodologies).

Brain imaging experiments are typically constructed as variations on a 'subtraction paradigm' (Friston et al. 1996, Overgaard 2004). That is, the persons in the scanner, known as 'subjects' in the lingo of the field (Roepstorff 2002), are exposed to highly controlled sets of stimuli known as 'conditions'. These are constructed so that they differ only in a few factors, typically one or two. The outcome of the experiment, the raw data, consists of a time series of files that depict three-dimensionally certain measurements from the brain. In the experiment discussed in the following pages, subjects had been placed in an MR scanner, which measures magnetic properties in tissue, and the scanner had been tuned to give an index of the amount of haemoglobin bound to oxygen in particular regions of the brain. This technique, known as Blood Oxygen Level Dependent Functional Magnetic Resonance Imaging or BOLD-fMRI, is a standard technique for cognitive activation studies. The underlying hypothesis is that when there is activity in a particular region of the brain, the vascular system somehow detects this and sends more blood to that region. This leads to an increase in the concentration of oxygen-haemoglobin complexes and hence an increase in the MR signal (Logothetis 2003).

In the actual data analysis, the raw data are first preprocessed. This means that in a number of black-boxed steps performed by a computer program, the images of the individual brains are rotated, pulled, pushed, squeezed and stretched till they come to fit with a 'standard brain' template that allows for comparison both between the subjects in an individual study and with other experiments (Beaulieu 2003, 2004; see also Cohn, this volume). Based on knowledge about when subjects were exposed to the different conditions, the investigator then constructs a model of the experiment. A computer program examines where in the brain this model may explain the data registered. The result of this is presented as an SPM, a statistical parametric map, which superimposes two types of information: on the one hand, an image of a 'standard' brain; on the other hand, a colour coding which illustrates how well the model explains the data in a particular part of the brain. The experimenter may choose different 'thresholds' for activation, i.e. decide how well the data should fit the model in order to be shown on the image. This thresholding may be compared with lowering the water level in an archipelago that has been completely flooded: at one level, nothing shows above the surface; when the water levels are lowered, isolated islands may occur; and as the water retracts, individual peaks may turn out to be part of larger, continuous land masses. This means that the modelling of the same data may be represented in many different ways, where some will not show any activation at all, others will show varying amounts of 'blobs' lighting up, while others again may paint the entire brain. A number of conventions provide the guidelines for how the images may be thresholded in different conditions, just as conventions govern how the statistical p-values are translated into a graded colour scale.

In effect, as in all other processes of scientific knowledge production, the initial raw data have, via procedures that are largely black-boxed, gone through parallel processes of reduction and amplification (Latour 1999). The data have been stripped of their individual context (measurement of a concrete person's brain at a particular time) and they have been transformed into a general framework that allows them to speak with some authority about general issues ('the brain' reacts to such stimuli in this particular way). As should be apparent from the description above, the images, which may to the uninitiated reader look like a 'snapshot' of the brain, should not in semiotic terms be considered realistic 'icons', governed by relations of similarity. They are better thought of as 'symbols', where a number of conventions govern the link between the image and that which it represents. Ideally, of course, the researcher hopes to establish with them a convincing indexical relationship, which points more or less directly to underlying brain processes.

Narrating the Blobs

With this knowledge at hand, let us return to the master. He had been given two series of statistical parametric maps, which showed forty-two horizontal slices through a standard brain superimposed with colour coded information indicating where the paradigm had caused activity (Figure 9.1). He was told that there were two main conditions in the experiment, and that the two images illustrated the areas where a particular condition caused an increase in activation. This was accompanied by the minimal specifications detailing technical aspects and the conventions followed and a table indicating the coordinates of the activated regions in a standard brain space.

The challenge was to try to identify what kind of experiment could have caused these images. The following is an edited transcription of his analysis

> This [figure 9.1] is a very clean result. There are very few blobs, and they are very nicely bilateral, so one is inclined to believe it. And then I were to think about, what the location might tell us ... These look very kind of visual. This is the parahippocampal cortex, I wanted to look things up, cause I can't remember coordinates very well, I mean, they are clearly not looking at faces, so this might be the parahippocampal place area so they might be looking at things that can be classified as places or have these sort of properties. The medial stuff, which is in retrosplenial, has been involved in retrieval of memory, and people with lesions in that area have problems with the retrieval. And the precuneus has also been involved in retrieval of memory tasks, but the one that I am particularly interested in, there is a study by Ray Dolan and others where people were shown degraded faces, and then they were told what it was [Dolan et al. 1997] ... so this area seems to be activated when you are looking at degraded images and you are using your prior knowledge to work out what they really are. And this actually does not only apply to vision, it also applies to stories ... So I would have to conclude that they were looking at some kind of degraded images and trying to work out what they were.
>
> Should I talk about the other one [figure 9.2]? One obviously wants to take them both into account, because obviously one problem with this type of analysis is that you can't distinguish between activations and inhibitions so that what you see here might be inhibitions in the opposite contrast. Who knows. Now this is very striking, particularly on this image. You have got all this activity running down the temporal lobe all the way down towards the temporal pole, particularly on the left, which make one think that it is very linguistic ... There are these areas here, which in fact I could not find on the table. They appear to be inferior frontal, probably not Broca's but [Brodmann's area] 45 or 47 ... they are probably something like Wernicke's area. And then there is this mysterious stuff in the medial frontal region, and I of course am interested in Theory of Mind but I think this is too high. The other option is that it is related to Marcus Raichle's default brain regions [Raichle et al. 2001], which tend to be more active during the control task, and the idea is that it deactivates whenever you have to do something difficult so perhaps one would argue that this task is the easier of the two, and I could not really talk more about giving this a sort of positive function. So in this case, I have to conclude that this looks sort of linguistic, and this is the thing you would expect if people were listening to narratives or reading narratives, which is very far away from the other task. And, yes that's all I have to say.

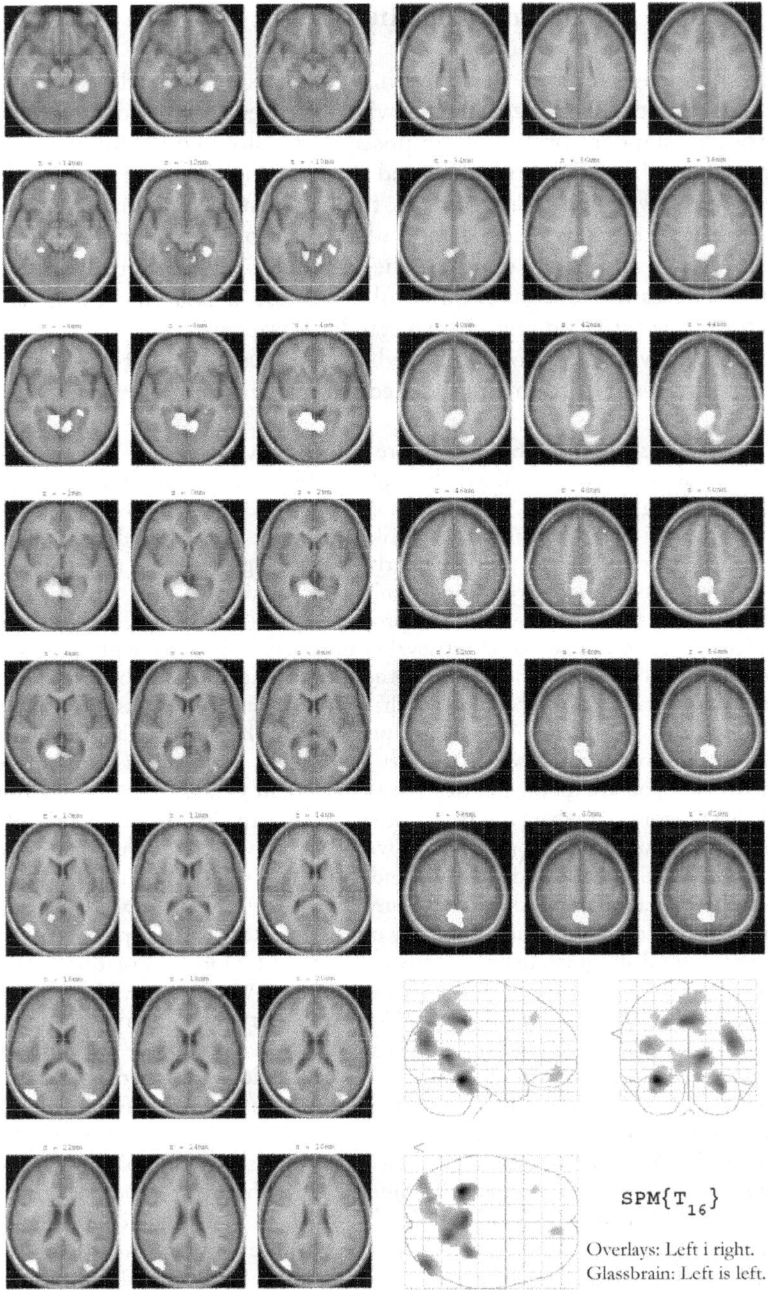

Figure 9.1 Statistical parametric mapping of increased activity caused by the first condition, superimposed on a standard brain.

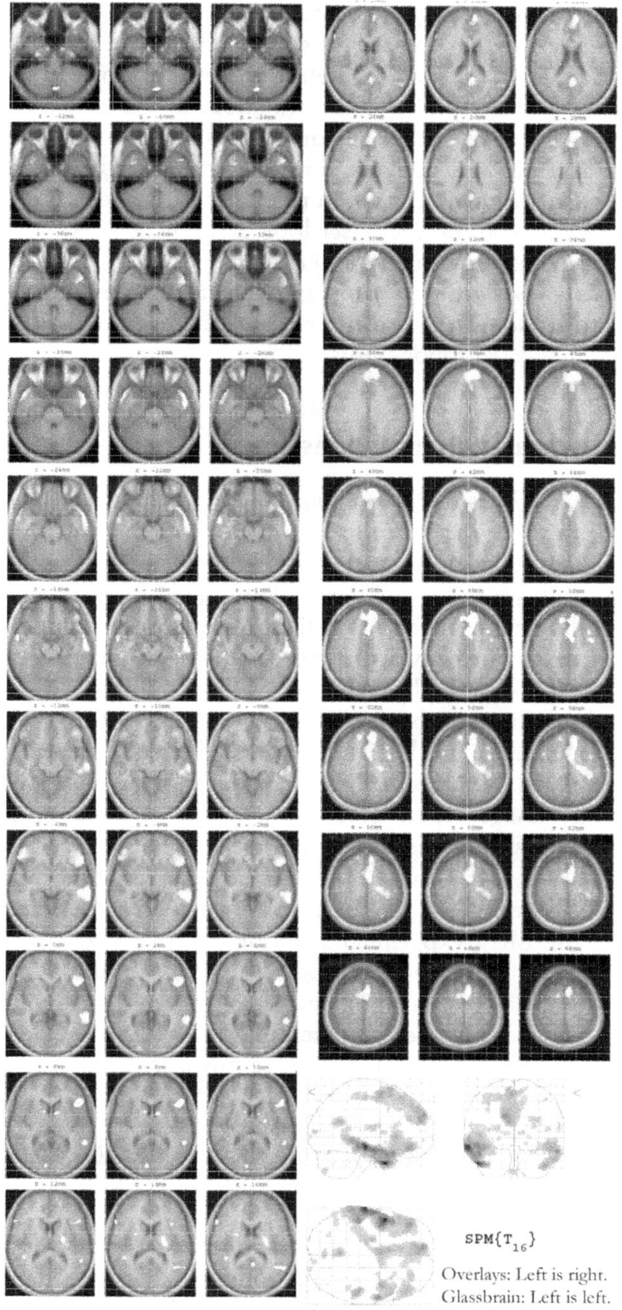

Figure 9.2 Statistical parametric mapping of increased activity caused by the second condition.

I mentioned earlier that we had set up this scenario as a tongue-in-cheek opening ritual to determine whether the master was worthy of the title. We unanimously decided that he was. In fact, his identification of one part of the experiment as processing of degraded visual information, the other part as narrative, proved two things. Firstly, that he could actually interpret brain images on the fly; secondly, that we had made some data that could be turned into a potentially interesting narrative. I shall return to that narrative in a little while, but before that, we need to take a closer look at a few aspects of his analysis. In parallel with the vignette that opened this article, it may be pertinent to describe it as a navigation in brainscape. Like the father pointing out significant features to the son, I will use quotes from his analysis to direct attention through the complicated topography.

Navigating the Brainscape

> *This is a very clean result. There are very few blobs, and they are very nicely bilateral, so one is inclined to believe it.*

One of the first things you learn when you enter a brain imaging laboratory as a novice, is that the colourful images of brains lighting up are very far from realistic photographs of the brain. They are rather to be seen as complicated graphs, the outcome of a set of complicated mathematical transformations that could have been done in a number of different ways. Most of these processes are black-boxed, and it is fairly difficult – indeed beyond the grasp of most researchers – to actually understand in all details these processes and their consequences. The images themselves, one learns, are therefore problematic entities; they look like solid facts, but, given the same data, they could have come to look very differently. How, then, to judge whether an image is interesting? One criterion is a fine balance between no activity and activity in all of the brain. Most experiments can be made to show such pictures, but they are difficult to interpret, indeed boring. The ideal is a few, nicely localised blobs, and if they are bilateral, it suggests that similar processes are going on in both hemispheres, something which it is difficult to obtain by chance. The metaphor 'clean' is therefore not only an aesthetic category, it also points to the character of the narrative to be unfolded.

> *These look very kind of visual … they might be looking at things that can be classified as places or have these sort of properties.*

How, then to find one's way through the brain? For decades, the 'brain mapping' field has tried to correlate mental functions to a concrete brain structure. Much early research was based on lesion studies and animal models, but during the last couple of decades, brain scanning techniques are increasingly used for that purpose. This has established a set of 'landmarks' in the brain, which are known to be involved in particular functions. The primary sensory cortices are among the least disputed; however, through mapping of sensory processes, it has also been possible to identify so-called 'higher' visual areas.

Some of these areas seem to be involved in things like motion, others in the perception of form or colour. People have tried to identify the difference between areas for faces and areas for places etc. (Epstein and Kanwisher 1998). This literature imposes on the brainscape a semantic overlay through which it becomes possible to 'see' in the images mental functions played out.

> *... so this area seems to be activated when you are looking at degraded images and you are using your prior knowledge to work out what they really are. And this actually does not only apply to vision, it also applies to stories ...*

However, the more one moves 'up' into the brain the more complicated this story of simple modularity seems to be, as is evidenced, for instance, from apparently 'visual' areas that may be activated by imaginations, or 'degradation' areas that appear to react to uncertainty, not only in vision but also in narratives etc. This makes the narrative navigation of the brainscape much more complicated. It is as if the basic vocabulary of modules-driven-by-the-senses in metaphorical and/or metonymic relations comes to 'mean' something more. One may therefore construct meaningful sentences like 'this area means "degraded image", but not only as an outside image, also an inside image will do the job' or 'this area means "faces" but not only as in seeing a face, on the outside also as in recalling a face from memory' (see O'Craven and Kanwisher 2000 for classic experiments of this type). Thereby the simplified modularity assumption becomes modified, as each module come to take on a certain polysemy, inscribed on it through an increasing set of experiments.

The more literature you know, the more experiments you may relate to, the more flexibility you have in actually interpreting the images, or, to put it slightly more cynically, the more you can allow yourself in having the data come to fit with the hypothesis, the better you can craft your argument in such a way that the reviewers will deem your paper to fit publications – your peers, who will be the gatekeepers to decide whether your data will be allowed to be inscribed into the polysemy of the meaning of brain regions.

> *I would have to conclude that they were looking at some kind of degraded images and trying to work out what they were.*

In this way, the 'semantics' of individual brain regions, established by previous experiments, allow one to transform a patterned network of brain activities into one narrative, which relates brain activity to human performance.

In our little ritual examination, this narrative was in no way constrained by the actual experiment; we shall return to that later. At this stage, the narrative mainly serves as a demonstration of how prior knowledge allows us to 'see', in the apparently random dots on a virtual representation of the brain, a certain narrative of human action and behaviour. If you compare Figure 9.3, which was the way the data became presented in the final article, with the relatively 'raw' data which our visitor was presented with (Figure 9.1) you will see that the final image has come to reflect the analysis. The first images, which represented the brain either as a set of slices or as a glass brain, and where colour intensity indiscriminately coded for how significant the activation was, have become transformed into a different representation. In the glass brain view, the colour coding now mainly highlights and groups together certain blobs into categories that each form semantic building blocks for a narrative. The rendering of the SPM on a standard brain has been perspectivised to facilitate one particular perspective on the data, enabled by a cut-through model of the brain.

This supports the analysis that we were dealing with activity in a number of regions, which together form an interpretable pattern. This 'style of representation' is indeed a deliberate choice; it transforms the raw data into what Ludwik Fleck called a '*Sinnbild*' or an 'ideogram', that is, an image which not only faithfully represents 'reality' but equally bears the mark of the 'thought style', the ideas and concepts, within which the image was formed (Fleck 1979). Images are arguments and, as will be apparent from the analysis of the next contrast, arguments should be tailored differently, depending on the use.

> *You have got all this activity running down the temporal lobe all the way down towards the temporal pole, particularly on the left, which make one think that it is very linguistic ...*

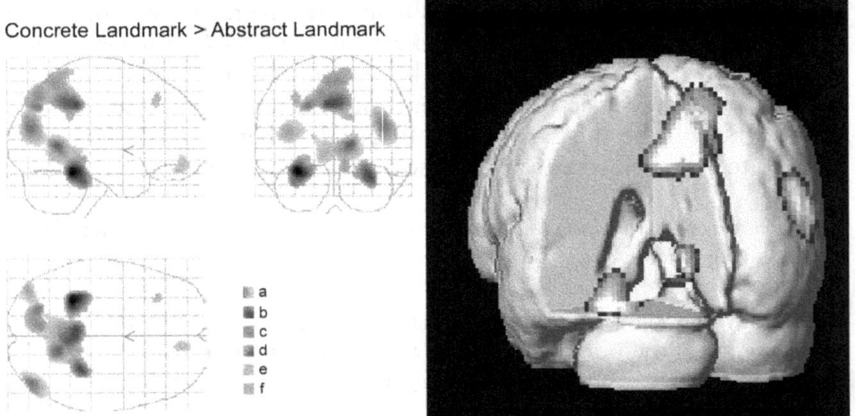

Figure 9.3 The final illustration of the activity caused by the first condition.

Also in this example the pattern of activity immediately attracts a particular interpretation: this is language. However, the link between the image and the narrative is configured slightly differently. This time it is not mainly driven by individual regions with individual semantics, it is rather the pattern as such, in the temporal cortex on the left, which almost shouts out 'language' to the informed reader. This does not require much further interpretation.

> *And then there is this mysterious stuff in the medial frontal region, and I of course am interested in Theory of Mind but I think this is too high. The other option is that it is related to Marcus Raichle's default brain regions, which tend to be more active during the control task.*

However, there is something strange lurking in these pictures – the 'mysterious stuff' that fails to fit into any of the obvious categories, an area one should perhaps rather try to avoid, by simply navigating around it, almost as when pointing out a treacherous ice floe in Torssukkattak. This area becomes personified by some of the researchers dealing in that region: Marcus Raichle, the grand master of PET-scanning, who has introduced the very controversial theory of 'default brain regions' (Raichle et al. 2001); the 'Theory of Mind crowd', who try to identify the neuronal correlates of social interaction in a related region (Gallagher and Frith 2003) – all in all a messy place that is difficult to enter, since all sorts of very different interpretations have to be weighed against each other, not through simple metonymic and metaphoric extensions of basic functions, but through radically contested basic semantics.

As you will see from a comparison between the first representation of the findings (Figure 9.2) and the published figure (Figure 9.4), the final image came to reflect this intuitive reading. The 'original' colour coding, where intensity codes for significance, has been maintained, and the data are presented as surface renderings, which highlight the activity 'running down the temporal lobe' and downplay the medial frontal stuff. Again, an ideogram, which this time almost shouts 'language', while not overemphasising 'the mysterious stuff' in the middle.

Crafting the Story

With this exposition of the analysis of a brain scan I have tried to demonstrate how particular blobs, seen through the eyes of an experienced reader, seem to drag along certain kinds of narratives. You have been in the same situation as our 'master-to-be', in that you have had no clues as to what made these images. I hope that this has allowed you to get a glimpse of a cognitive mapping within the field of brain imaging. It is a mapping between blobs and semantics, which allows for an unfolding of certain narratives. In this navigation of the brainscape, certain features stand out as facts: 'these look very kind of visual', 'it is very linguistic', these couplings have a certain facticity to them. They are 'facts' in the sense of Ludwik Fleck – *denkkollektives wiederstandsaviso*, signs of resistance to the thought community – that, although not quite as stable as the ice floes in Torssukkattak, present obstacles to free navigation (Fleck 1979; see discussion in Roepstorff 2004).

> *So in this case, I have to conclude that this looks sort of linguistic, and this is the thing you would expect if people were listening to narratives or reading narratives, which is very far away from the other task.*

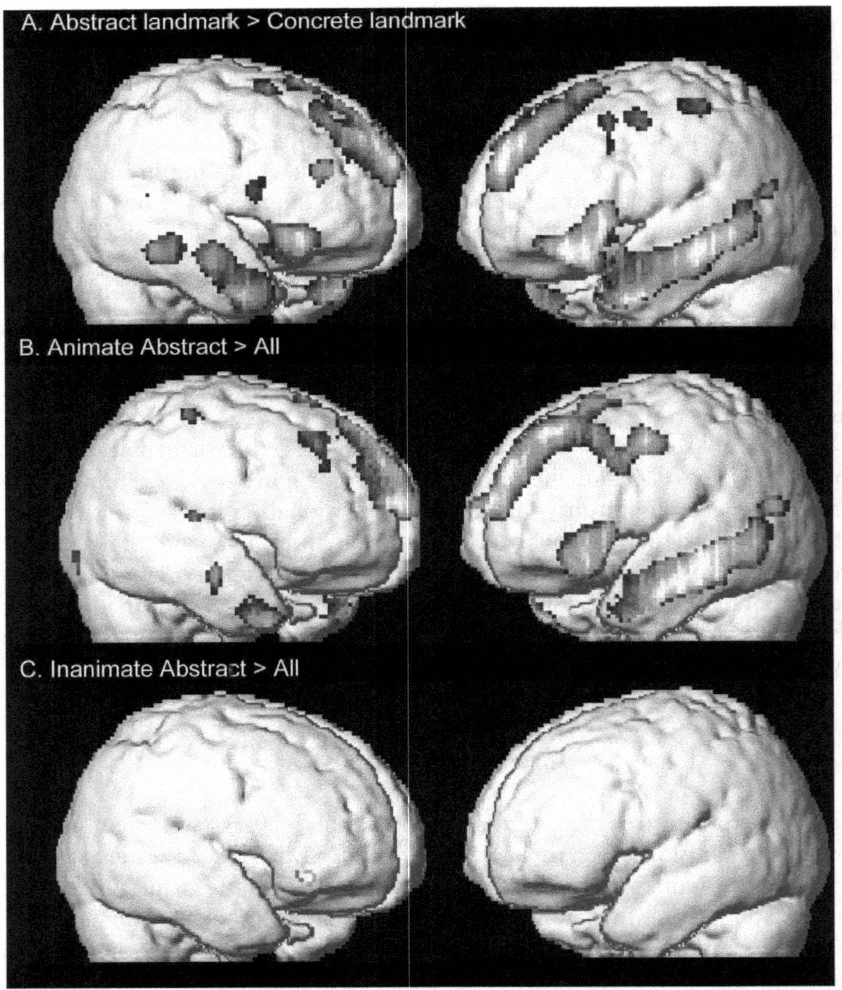

Figure 9.4 The final illustration of the activity caused by the second condition.

At this stage in our initiation ritual the 'true' meaning of the images was exposed. The experiment was an attempt at studying how words embedded in simple sentences could be made to imbue different meanings. Very briefly, during the part of the experiment that looked 'visual', the persons in the scanner heard or read sentences of the type 'the man enters the forest' or , 'the path enters the forest', that is, simple motion constructions with an animate or an inanimate grammatical subject and concrete nouns in the prepositional construction. During the part of the experiment that looked 'sort of linguistic', people heard or read sentences like 'the man enters the sorrow', or the slightly obscure 'the path enters the sorrow', that is, motion constructions with an animate or an inanimate grammatical subject and abstract nouns in the propositional construction (Wallentin et al. 2005).

The fact that the concrete sentences generated brain activations that in themselves 'looked very kind of visual', allowed the researcher, in the analysis and the writing up of the story, to embark on one particular narrative trajectory through the brainscape. The resulting article could confidently claim that: 'These findings support a model of language where the understanding of spatial semantic content emerges from the recruitment of brain regions involved in non-linguistic spatial processing.' Mikkel Wallentin, the first author of the paper, had indeed designed the experiment to examine and falsify a hypothesis of an activation of 'non-linguistic' regions by language, so both from a Popperian perspective and from a constructivist perspective on knowledge production, the experiment was a success.

In choosing this interpretation, the final article settled on a relatively safe navigation. It almost completely bypassed 'the mysterious stuff in the medial prefrontal region' and the complicated questions involved in taking both activations into account at the same time. Not that Wallentin did not want to chart these waters; however, after long discussions, we decided to leave those brainscapes for later, for a time when there were enough facts floating around to allow us to be somewhat more qualified to answer the 'who knows' of the relation between activation and deactivation, between context and content.

Conclusion: When Knowing Becomes Seeing

When I began writing this chapter, memories of Torssukkattak Icefjord kept pressing themselves to the foreground, while I thought I was writing about brain scans. I therefore decided to let them write themselves into the chapter, not really knowing what they were going to do there. But in this post-hoc analysis, they may have done so for very good reasons. I think that there are at least two levels of metaphorical connections.

The first and most obvious involves seeing and learning to see. I hope that the narrative has demonstrated convincingly that learning to see a brain image is a process which involves knowing, and that it unfolds in a social scenario where significant features, through concrete others or through others by the proxy of scientific literature, are being pointed out and imbued with meaning. Just like learning to sail through ice-filled waters, this process unfolds in a social setting where significant features are pointed out. This social interaction creates joint fields of attention, which serve to support interpretation (which narratives can be generated and sustained?) and action (which steps to take next, in data analysis and experimental designs?). This suggests that knowledge serves as a necessary background for seeing or, to put it slightly differently, that effective seeing – seeing that may be connected to action – appears to some extent conceptual. In the first analysis, the interrelation of knowing and seeing may appear more prominent in the brain imaging setting, where 'knowing' explicitly appears a necessary prerequisite for 'seeing', as in 'this looks very visual'. In contrast, the silent ice-navigation scenario could be taken to suggest a more tacit mode of knowledge (Polanyi 1964). However, recent discussions in the philosophy of cognition may suggest that such difference is one of degree rather than one of kind.

In a recent comprehensive review, Alva Noë (2004) convincingly argues for an enactive understanding, which grounds both perception and cognition in a joint sensory-motor substratum, modified by experience and both prompted and stabilised by external cues. This line of argumentation, which holds much promise for an anthropological analysis, appears compatible with the 'ingoldian position' (Ingold 2000) known to most anthropologists, but it is better grounded in, and in exchange, with recent developments in cognitive science and philosophy. It allows one to identify how enskilled sensitivity to perceptual affordances, irrespective of apparent differences in the mode of communication, develops competences that are at the same time cognitive and practical. It is remarkable here that in the two cases discussed, the enskilled vision appears to enable an identification of agency. An understanding of agency, of ice floes or of brain regions, is crucial both for navigating ice-filled waters and for navigating brains, since it allows one to explore novel routes no matter whether they are practical (getting from A to B) or epistemic (understanding why and how one gets there). That agency is pivotal also in practical and epistemic processes suggests an important epistemic extension to Gell's wonderful anthropological theory of art (Gell 1998). Epistemic processes, such as found in skilled vision, involve a stipulation of indices that allows for an identification of agency, where the 'index of agency' (ibid., 66) is non-human. This suggests links between aesthetics and epistemics, which, however, are beyond the scope of this chapter to explore further.

At a different level, there may also be a more metaphorical connection at stake between the two cases. Perhaps this whole process of 'navigating the brainscape', of charting regions and drafting narratives of them, bears some structural similarity to sailing in ice-filled waters. In this instance, however, both the fix-points and the obstacles are facts, established through other experiments, solidified through other narratives. These facts have a very strong social dimension to them. They are facts in Fleck's sense, signs of resistance to a thought collective. In navigating them, that is, mapping them and thereby drafting new interpretations of them, one has to take into account not only the 'intrinsic nature' they seem to reveal in the actual experiment, but also the already established meanings inscribed on them. This sets limits to the type of interpretations, the types of narratives that will stand a chance of being believed. In this sense, knowing how to see, and, as importantly, knowing how the other transforms seeing into knowing is therefore imperative for being a proper member of the brain imaging community. This renders the findings with a double nature, they appear at once solidly given and socially fluid, factishes, in Bruno Latour's wording (Latour 1999; see also discussion in Roepstorff and Bubandt 2003). Brain imaging facts are therefore complicated entities, not only to the anthropologist trying to describe them, but also to the burgeoning scientist trying to produce them. In this chapter I have also, as a somewhat hidden agenda, tried to argue that both in the understanding of the 'nature of facts' and in the production of 'stable facts', these two perspectives – the construction and the deconstruction – may benefit from going hand in hand (Roepstorff 1999).

Acknowledgements

This research was supported by grants from the Danish National Research Foundation and from the Danish Research Council for Humanities. Figures were produced by Mikkel Wallentin, who, as always, also provided highly useful comments to an earlier version of this manuscript, as did the anonymous reviewer.

References

Beaulieu, A. 2003. 'Brain, Maps and the New Territory of Psychology', *Theory & Psychology* 13: 561–68.

——— 2004. 'From Brainbank to Database: The Informational Turn in the Study of the Brain', *Studies in History and Philosophy of Science Part C: Studies in History and Philosophy of Biological and Biomedical Sciences* 35: 367–90.

Dolan, R.J., G.R. Fink, E. Rolls, M. Booth, A. Holmes, R.S. Frackowiak and K.J. Friston, 1997. 'How the Brain Learns to See Objects and Faces in an Impoverished Context', *Nature* 389: 596–99.

Epstein, R. and N. Kanwisher, 1998. 'A Cortical Representation of the Local Visual Environment', *Nature* 392: 598–601.

Fleck, L. 1979. *Genesis and Development of a Scientific Fact*. Chicago: Chicago University Press.

Frackowiak, R.S. et al., ed. 2004. *Human Brain Function*. London: Academic Press.

Friston, K.J., C.J. Price, P. Fletcher, C. Moore, R.S. Frackowiak, and R.J. Dolan, 1996. 'The Trouble with Cognitive Subtraction', *Neuroimage* 4: 97–104.

Gallagher, H.L. and C.D. Frith, 2003. 'Functional Imaging of "Theory of Mind"', *Trends in Cognitive Sciences* 7: 77–83.

Gell, A. 1998. *Art and Agency. An Anthropological Theory.* Oxford: Clarendon Press.

Gibson, J. 1979. *The Ecological Approach to Visual Perception.* Boston: Houghton Mifflin.

Ingold, T. 2000. *The Perception of the Environment.* London: Routledge.

—— 2001. 'From the Transmission of Representations to the Education of Attention', in *The Debated Mind: Evolutionary Psychology versus Ethnography*, ed. H. Whitehouse. Oxford: Berg, 113–53.

—— 2003. 'Three in One', in *Imagining Nature*, eds. A. Roepstorff, N. Bubandt and K. Kull. Aarhus: Aarhus University Press: 40–55.

Latour, B. 1999. *Pandora's Hope: Essays on the Reality of Science Studies.* Cambridge, Mass.: Harvard University Press.

Logothetis, N.K. 2003. 'The Underpinnings of the BOLD Functional Magnetic Resonance Imaging Signal', *Journal of Neuroscience* 23: 3963–71.

Nöe, A. 2004. *Action in Perception.* Cambridge, Mass.: MIT Press.

O'Craven, K.M. and N. Kanwisher, 2000. 'Mental Imagery of Faces and Places Activates Corresponding Stimulus-Specific Brain Regions', *Journal of Cognitive Neuroscience* 12: 1013–23.

Overgaard, M. 2004. 'Confounding Factors in Contrastive Analysis', *Synthese* 141: 217–31.

Pálsson, G. 1994. 'Enskilment at Sea', *Man* 29: 901–27.

—— 2000. '"Finding One's Sea Legs": Learning, the Process of Enskilment, and Integrating Fishers and Their Knowledge Into Fisheries Science and Management', in *Finding Our Sea Legs: Linking Fishery People and Their Knowledge with Science and Management*, eds. B. Neis, and L. Felt. St. Johns: ISER Books, 24–33.

Polanyi, M. 1964. *The Tacit Dimension.* New York: Anchor Books.

Raichle, M.E., A.M. Macleod, A.Z. Snyder, W.J. Powers, D.A.Gusnard and G.L. Shulman, 2001. 'A Default Mode of Brain Function', *Proceedings of the National Academy of Sciences of the United States of America* 98: 676–82.

Roepstorff, A. 1999. 'Deconstructing Social Constructionism', *FOLK, Journal of the Danish Ethnographic Society* 41: 139–54.

—— 2002. 'Transforming Subjects into Objectivity. An Ethnography of Knowledge in a Brain Imaging Laboratory', *FOLK, Journal of the Danish Ethnographic Society* 44: 145–70

—— 2003. 'Clashing Cosmologies. Contrasting Knowledges in the Greenlandic Fishery', in *Imagining Nature. Practices of Cosmology and Identity*, eds. A. Roepstorff, N. Bubandt and K. Kull. Aarhus: Aarhus University Press, 117–42.

—— 2004. 'Mapping Brain Mappers: an Ethnographic Coda', in *Human Brain Function*, 2nd edn., eds. R.S. Frackowiak et al. Elsevier: 1105–17.

Roepstorff, A. and N Bubandt, 2003. 'Introduction: The Critique of Culture and the Plurality of Nature', in *Imagining Nature. Practices of Cosmology and Identity*, eds. A. Roepstorff, N. Bubandt and K. Kull. Aarhus: Aarhus University Press, 9–31.

Wallentin, M., S. Østergaard, T. Lund, L. Østergaard and A. Roepstorff, 2005. 'Concrete Spatial Language. See What I Mean?', *Brain and Language* 92: 221–33.

Epilogue

Envisioning Skills: Insight, Hindsight, and Second Sight

Michael Herzfeld

There is, Cristina Grasseni suggests, a besetting embarrassment about the centrality of the visual in anthropology; we see, we report on what we observe, but we do not like the implications of that commitment. It is time, she says, to do something about this unhelpful paradox. And so the authors in this volume recuperate the centrality of vision in anthropological understanding. Their effort is less one of discovering a new emphasis for the discipline as of forcing awareness of an entailment already engaged. To have thus reconfigured the discipline's mode of attention is no small achievement, and in itself it speaks to core issues in the essays gathered here: the relationship between habit and attention, and the relative invisibility of a visual capacity. Such is the logic of Poe's purloined letter: it is always, so to speak, in full view. Recovering awareness of its presence serves the historically and conceptually definitional anthropological mission of denaturalising 'common sense'.

In precisely this spirit, the authors draw on the inherently visualist basis of a central anthropological concern by introducing a strongly comparative focus. Theirs is not the old systemic comparativism of structural functionalism, but a willingness to offer hitherto unthinkable juxtapositions, including some that force anthropology to confront itself as a key *comparandum*. The various chapters progressively reveal the difficulty of the task these authors have thereby set themselves. Vision is not only the authoritative and self-conscious activity that characterises surveillance and invites charges of 'visualism' (Fabian 1983; Goody 1977). It is also a learned capacity. As such, it is thoroughly cultural, requiring ethnographic specificity in consideration of its appearances everywhere, from Yukhagir hunters' techniques to medical brain scanning. Sight is less an exercise of power as such than an activity through which certain social actors find the materials for the maintenance of that power.

Several authors here explicitly modulate the recent critiques of visualism in anthropology by repositioning the links between sight and power. This rearguard action entails a risk, less that of ignoring the entailment of sight-based skills in hierarchical arrangements of power – the authors clearly recognise this – than in potentially encouraging the wilful evasion of these political realities. Indeed, the serious political implications of the often rich and always suggestive historical and ethnographic materials discussed here sometimes seem analytically attenuated. Yet it is in the political dynamics of knowedge production and transmission that we can most clearly reap the advantages of 'seeing' vision as a trained activity – Gibson's 'education of attention'. Education is always about access to knowledge; training also sometimes occludes as much as it reveals. Consequently, the cognitivist tendency in some of the arguments advanced here does not so much defeat as confirm Fabian's (1983) central critique, one aspect of which is to show that formal cognitive analysis – appropriately rejected in its formalist guise by, for example, Ronzon, even as he seeks to salvage its more useful implications –systematically occludes the enabling political conditions of its own academic authority. Fabian's original critique is in fact vital to the arguments advanced in this book.

The loss of political focus – our loss of political vision – is a consequence, not of the attempt to recover vision for the discipline, but of a common tendency to assume that training – or apprenticeship, to emphasise its social aspects – is necessarily about the transmission of instrumental knowledge. This assumption mistakes technique for epistemology. We see confirmed here, however, that apprenticeship is at least as likely to entail the transmission of conventional attitudes as a specific set of craft procedures. Those attitudes, moreover, provide handles for the more powerful to retain control over interpretation and evaluation as well as the acquisition of knowledge as such; artisans sometimes actively try to *prevent* their apprentices from directly learning the secrets of the trade (see, for example, Herzfeld 2004).

Learning how to see is partly a matter of absorbing a taxonomy – which then serves as a grid, limiting as well as enabling access to information. Classification is in this sense, as Fabian points out, a highly political *and* a highly visual activity – which is precisely why it has retained such an important position in anthropology. Combining the Gramscian view of common sense as an effect of hegemony with Mary Douglas's (1966, 1986) insights into the relationship between social structure (the distribution of power) and taxonomy, we see how vision is culturally shaped and controlled to produce a sense of an unchanging *doxa* embedded in a social as well as physical landscape (Bourdieu 1977).

In the process, the authors of these essays are doing something that Fabian's critique demands: examining the visual activity of various social actors, including anthropologists themselves, in order to see how ways of seeing can be shaped to serve particular interests. Bleichmar, for example, draws extremely useful links between colonialism and particular ways of visualising, drawing out the play between images of nature and of human variety and especially highlighting the absences that paradoxically buttress the confident colonial sense of knowledge that is both replete and controlled. The Linnaean scheme of natural classification also 'naturalized' a hierarchy of human kinds (see Herzfeld 1987: 96–98; Hodgen 1964: 425–26). Bleichmar has extended this insight, showing how the visual skills of intellectuals served to reinforce a worldview that supported the colonial project. In effect, it 'en-iconised' human physical features as representations of mental traits, much as later collections of folklore were used to 'entextualise' social groups (see especially Raheja 1996). Such analyses undermine the assumption that intellectual labour somehow stands free of embodied understanding.

Others here have been less explicit in addressing the politics of vision, but it is worth drawing out those implications as well. Grasseni, for example, engages a fundamentally political theme. She shows how types of expertise can be inculcated through the play activity of herders' children, in which we find a suggestively heavy overlap, temporal as well as conceptual, with the serious business of classifying livestock. She also recognises how the values thus learned, and those who learn them, are drawn into a hierarchy that spreads far beyond any local or even national community through what, in her introductory essay, she calls 'local-global dynamics'.

This is not merely a recovery of vision for anthropology. It fills a more serious lacuna, by showing how sight is socially and culturally managed. That is the force of Grasseni's identification of the dual sense of vision, as physical sight and as worldview, and it allows us to link the *practice* of seeing as a skill to the ideological and intellectual assumptions that it expresses and reproduces. Such an approach offers a grasp of the political dynamics of knowledge creation, including, decisively, our own. It would be a pity were readers to miss this crucial linkage, with its attendant refutation of the stereotype of anthropology as obsessively engaged only with the local, the marginal and the trivial, condemned to reproduce iconically its own irrelevance to the world at large.

The political dimension is crucial for two particular reasons. The first of these is that the comparative project is inherently political in itself. As I argued some years ago, inserting anthropology as a cultural object into any comparative effort will raise issues of the political constitution of the discipline itself; in my case, the comparison was with Greece, a nation-state whose existence resembled that of the discipline in that both emerged from colonialism's concern with clear boundaries and their ideological legitimation (Herzfeld 1987). While Willerslev's attempt to do something similar here must rely on both his other publications on Yukhagir ethnography and on his readers' presumed knowledge of the social life of anthropology, he does begin to turn the critical searchlight back onto anthropological practice, revealing it as profoundly and necessarily visual in important respects.

That is valuable in itself. A more robust acknowledgement of these Siberian hunters as theorists might nevertheless have still further reduced the distance between ethnographer and informant, and so led to a critical assessment of why the role of vision for both hunter and anthropologist cannot be reduced to the visualist conventions of anthropological formalisms. Do we know, for example, that Yukhagir experience vision exactly as Merleau-Ponty assumes all humans do? If experience transcends cultural categories, Willerslev here provides even stronger support for Fabian's argument against the priority of 'visualist' – note, *not* 'visual' – categories. Both hunting and theorising are social practices, and thus belong, at least in this sense, to an order of mutually comparable activities.

The other dimension of the politics of knowledge that unites these essays in at least an implicit sense lies in the recognition of a 'global hierarchy of value' (Herzfeld 2004 and Grasseni, this volume). This is the effect of those cultural forces that have insidiously but forcefully replaced the more overt control mechanisms of colonial rule, thereby completing the logic, first identified by Ernest Gellner (1983: 000), of the shift in the creation of nation-states from face-to-face (or what in semiotics are called *indexical*) relations to relations based on presumed commonalities (*iconic* relations); now culture, globalised as 'heritage', aestheticises all but the crudest and most bulky girders of the old military and economic forms of domination, redirecting local habits of embodiment to the fulfilment of Fordist or Taylorist quotas and logics and recasting the enchantment of lived experience as productive efficiency and precision (e.g., Blum 2000; see also Saunders, this volume) and the immediacy of social relations as membership in a uniform 'culture'. Even the claim that modern culture permits heterogeneity overlooks the extent to which 'individualism' is seen as a *common* property of the largely Western (or Western-trained) global elite, in which actual demonstrations of individuality risk marginalising particular social actors and groups as eccentrics or troublemakers. This is why most medical practitioners would, at least in public, increasingly resist Cohn's identification of the artistic element in what they do; the implication, once imbued with the aura of a mystical power, has instead become that of a creativity that both escapes and defies the rule of reason and therefore deserves no political authority in the modern, scientific world.

The force of this global hierarchy appears with particular and dreadful clarity in the effects of contesting it. Skilled workers who complain about the conditions of modern labour find themselves 'deskilled', their protests a confirmation – from the perspective of those in power – of their unsuitability for higher status (e.g., Blum 2000). Digitalisation may, as Cohn notes, also serve to dethrone such Cartesian logics, but the implication of both his and Roepstorff's contributions seems to be that in practice medical staff workers are instead also being 'deskilled', their openly expressed creativity a barrier to their advancement in a scientistic universe of knowledge production. More obviously, perhaps, and in a process that has clearer association with the structure of class relations in the industrialised world, artisans whose visual skills in many cultures centrally entail 'stealing with their eyes' ensure the transmission, not only of crafts as socially demeaning as they are admired for their picturesqueness, but of an association with aggression and sly cunning and a hostility to the use of language that debars them from any recognition of their intellectual capacities. They are trapped in the exaltation of 'tradition', whereby the price of approbation is surrender to the power of those who bestow it (Herzfeld 2004).

While these dynamics are not entirely ineluctable, escape usually entails accepting the principles on which they are based. One may make choices, but these choices themselves form part of larger, uneven distributions of power. Gunn, for example, usefully speaks of the embodied practices of artists as resisting institutionalisation; a consequence of such resistance, however, and one insufficiently acknowledged in the rather romanticising literature on resistance as a social phenomenon (notably Scott 1985; see Abu-Lughod 1990), is that it marks artists as, again, eccentrics or troublemakers and perpetually threatens to turn their principled non-conformism against them, enhancing its market value mostly to the benefit of highly successful entrepreneurs while depreciating the artists' ability to define their personal status outside their own specialised realm.

The training of visual skills – whether of artists, artisans, medical technicians or cattle herders – sustains the force of hierarchy by placing these social actors at various degrees of distance from a pinnacle defined, in the Cartesian scheme of power inherited from colonialism, by the exercise of pure ratiocination. Here, in fact, the advocates of a renewed emphasis on vision again find themselves in agreement with the critics of visualism, because, as Cohn says, 'the very idea of knowledge is usually assumed to be solely concerned with rational thought, conscious awareness, and with knowing that one knows something', and this conflicts with the recognition of knowledge as embedded in a skilled vision that is not – and in some cases must never be – rendered explicit. Indeed, for those who 'steal with their eyes' the absence of speech signifies a 'counter-cultural' skill, in which momentary success nonetheless spells long-term failure and exclusion. Class, classification and pedagogy merge here: the very affirmation that some skills cannot be learned in the classroom also locates their possessors in a system of class.

I have mentioned the shift from indexical relations of mutual knowledge to the entailment of entire populations in the iconic identification of 'culture'. The Peircean terminology offers a further advantage: Peirce's own central concern with *abduction*, the process of recovering knowledge by hindsight, is elegantly transmuted here into a tool of social analysis by Saunders. It neatly relieves us of one burden of the Cartesian logic that undergirds the global hierarchy of value: that most people find it hard not to think of intellectual activity, notably including reading and writing, as radically different from, and superior to, the manual skills more traditionally associated with artisanship. This position, as Cohn points out, entails the further assumption that intellectual labour is self-aware. It is a testimony to the successful implantation of hierarchical perspectives in an increasingly global 'common sense'. (If you are self-aware, you exercise control; if you wear tight, relatively short clothes, your body can function as an efficient machine, and this in turn justifies your claims to *imperium*, as the Linnaean taxonomy implies.) The carriers of this attitude are the powerful whose interests it serves, and who ironically do not recognise themselves as having an ideology at all. As Bleichmar's insight into reading as a form of training demonstrates, however, it is possible to reconstruct the inculcation of such a dominant perspective into those who think that they have invented reason and that they now control it.

The link between seeing and knowledge – etymologically embedded in many European languages, but obscured by a definitively colonialist (Rabinow 1989) urge to separate mind from body – recuperates the Sanskrit root (*viddhya*; cf. Thai *witthayaa*) that gives us both *vision* (and *video*) on the one hand and *Wissenschaft* (and *wit*) on the other. To abduce that connection between the *sensate* and the *sensual* now, via the defamiliarising devices of ethnographic comparison, is also therefore to recover a Vichian political history of concepts. This history recognises a perception that does not begin with abstract ratiocination, does not organise data according to a preconceived plan, but takes advantage of the sense of the suggestively named sense of *déjà vu* that informs many of the conceptual practices discussed in these pages.

I emphasise the Peircean terminology partly in order to recognise both its skilful application here and the dangers that could attend its misuse. Speaking of icons as though they were emblems, for example, is confusing; reducing all iconicity to the visual is inaccurate; and treating icons as things rather than characteristic uses (see Eco 1976) is merely reductionist. Thus, while Ronzon describes 'gay icons' in rich detail, they may actually be more symbolic or emblematic than iconic in the strict Peircean sense; the conversations Ronzon reports suggest as much. There may also be elements of both modalities. Distinguishing between them would show even more clearly how the images in question are made to serve a localised and fractious politics of cultural identity.

Such perceptual slippages are nonetheless hard to avoid, in part because they correspond to social experience. Herein lies the force of iconicity as a rhetorical device, as particularly exemplified by the way in which the powerful appropriate the idea of a collective 'culture': we are all alike, 'therefore' we should accept a common authority, which then displaces the untidiness of feuding, gossip and ritual manipulation. Law and regulation appear, abductively, to reproduce conceptual and perceptual order – which is another way of stating part of Douglas's (1966) celebrated thesis that pollution is 'matter out of place', but recasting it as a critique of the politics of perception. Thus, Turnbull speaks of 'iconic examples of good design', merging the sense of *recognisability* that characterises iconic relations with the emblematic or exemplary status that permits standardisation and efficiency. (The map of the London Underground, for example, is indeed an 'iconic example of good design' – but it is iconic in *both* senses, since visitors to London see it as both a portrait of the system it purports to represent and as an emblem – and perhaps also as an icon – of the kind of efficiency that is associated with the 'Tube'.) And again, in line with what I have just said about Saunders's chapter, Turnbull shows precisely how the impression of pure iconicity allows planners to represent a thoroughly disordered, hit-or-miss process of accumulation through time to appear instead as an atemporal order of remarkable perfection.

Putting terminology into question, however nominalistic, is useful here because it emphasises how easily relations of resemblance (visual or otherwise) become naturalised, forcing us to reconstruct the abductive processes whereby we recover the logic that led to that original intuition. We can identify similar conceptual processes among our informants; Willerslev's description of how the Yukhagir conceive of the *ayibii* suggests a process of abduction from a notion of common form to the specific resemblance between the hunter and his prey. Nor is abduction antithetical to modernity: the Texan oil tycoons described by Marcus (1992) retrospectively discover family resemblances – his 'dynastic uncanny' – that then appear to justify patrimonial succession as forcefully as do Greek islanders' post-partum recognitions of psychological family likeness (Vernier 1991). The operation of such retrospective second sight also extends to the world of organisation: the force of a document such as the London Underground map lies partly in the fact that it can be infinitely reproduced, reinforcing the sense of natural resemblance to which travellers experiences of reality are then calibrated as something always-already present in their lives.

Turnbull's analysis is exemplary in revealing these aleatory properties in what is abductively recognised as systemic activity. Such muddling through characterises all social life (de Certeau 1984; Reed-Danahay 1996; Scott 1998); Turnbull reminds us that planners, no less than their customers, are social beings. The presumed iconicity of the Underground map and the post hoc regularity of Chartres Cathedral are thus perfect illustrations of how culturally enforced conventions contribute to a perception of similarity and systematicity, rendering social chaos as cultural order. The conversion of ad hoc process into post hoc system occurs through what Turnbull appropriately calls 'performance', a process that may render palatable, even comforting, a structure of surveillance or regimentation.

Such structural inventions typically include the master plans of cities such as Le Corbusier's Chandigarh and Hausmann's Paris. Those designs, examples of what James C. Scott (1998) calls 'high-modernism', exalt abstract logic over lived experience. They also generate incredible suffering; weak populations, unable to resist such experiments in improved living, must fend for themselves. Most nevertheless manage to muddle through precisely because the system ignores their existence. This capacity compels comparison with the planners' actions; it is a rickety scaffolding that undergirds their claims to reason and permanence.

Formal, precise terminology has one practical advantage. It offers distance from the common sense that constitutes our own *habitus*. It thereby helps us understand why vision has been so thoroughly 'backgrounded' (Douglas 1975) in anthropological writing. We see because we are sufficiently distanced from what we see, as Merleau-Ponty points out (see Willerslev, this volume), but also because, ipso facto, we can generally describe what we see more easily than what we smell or taste.

Ronzon's ethnography suggests a productive further avenue: as we listen to speech about vision, recognising the apparent interdependence of the two modalities, we might find in the transvestites' conversations some clues to the ways in which anthropologists – similarly proud of their marginality – train each other to find aesthetic pleasure (the exotic, even if that is no longer fashionable, and the structured, which is even less so) in the social and cultural arrangements they encounter in the course of fieldwork. Ronzon does not tell us *how* the transvestites translate their comments into vision, but here we can turn to Roepstorff's splendid predication of the indexical signing of fishermen on a world of dangerous experience on the similarly 'inchoate' (Fernandez 1974) nudgings and mutterings of the apprentice medical staff reading their scans. it is clear from Ronzon's detailed reporting that his informants were equally adept at reading cues – indeed, that is partly why they were initially impatient, like many skilled informants, with his apparent inability to understand everything that was happening.

We may similarly probe the apparently direct contradiction between the verbally reproducible accessibility of vision in everyday life and the curiously self-concealing, taken-for-granted status of vision in anthropology itself. Anthropological training is often inchoate; explicit instruction raises suspicions of the betrayal of craft (see Rabinow 1977). We try to teach methods, but we always complain about how difficult it is. What Bleichmar calls the *je ne sais quoi* of the abductive process suggests the primacy of experience: you 'can't actually teach someone to be a good fieldworker', so it is said, because, as Roepstorff acknowledges, knowing is as often the prerequisite of seeing as seeing is of knowing. Needham (1972: 237–38) long ago acknowledged the physicality of writing: it appears to direct thought rather than be directed by it. If in Gunn's portrayal of David we see a man becoming part of a place, or if place can even consume the artist who becomes too attached to it (Willerslev, this volume), it is only after the fact that we as social actors can appreciate the methods that, we assure ourselves, were forming in our heads.

Methods are important, even in the absence of a conviction that they follow some inherently irreducible logic. The comparativist insertion of anthropology into its own gaze perhaps echoes the acquisition of new skills in ethnographic analysis: photography, videotaping and its reuse in reflexive exercises with informants, even, perhaps, some of the less reductionist forms of computer simulation. The medical scanning described by Cohn and Roepstorff offer especially strong models with which to compare anthropological forms of representation (the assumption that videotapes are somehow more 'real' than verbal descriptions offers one obvious path of critique), especially when mediated by Gunn's analysis of artists' relations with the physical world. If seeing requires distance, the *regard éloigné* (Lévi-Strauss 1983) of the anthropologist is also the prerequisite of what constitutes the act of ethnographic research – local intimacy, which may open up the encompassing society's sense of its more private cultural secrets (Herzfeld 2005). Anthropologists in the field frequently find their more 'inquisitive' recording technology viewed with suspicion; such tools are iconic of equipment used by police officers, intrusive journalists and spies. (I also sense that video cameras are more often tolerated than tape recorders; this is perhaps less for reasons of a lingering iconicity than because different machines evoke different indexical links – tape recorders evoke the police, but camcorders are clearly a family item in this consumerist age.)

Because sight offers natural-seeming signs, it easily obviates or subverts analysis, as Bleichmar suggests. We know *by* seeing; as Roepstorff notes, seeing *is* knowing, or at least we experience it as such even though knowing may well be a precondition for sight. That is why detailed ethnography is so important: vivid verbal depiction creates the illusion of shared vision, allowing the reader to grasp materially what otherwise could only be conveyed abstractly, and also provides plenty of material to work critically against one's own cultural expectations. Ronzon's ethnography, for example, richly evokes both vision and hearing as these undermine his own prior assumptions about the nature of beauty; the conversations race along, and we begin to perceive others through the eyes, as it were, of his interlocutors. Ultimately, then, his plea for a cognitive understanding of what he describes, far from reproducing the mechanistic object of Fabian's critique, is persuasive in that it follows rather than leads the ethnography.

This takes me back to the key metaphor that Saunders adduces: the 'CT suite' as a place of 'following'. Not only is there hierarchy, a political arena with leaders and followers clearly role-identified and partially deployed in the unequal idiom of pedagogical relations. There is also logical following: the analytic processes are abductive, working back from apparently random and messy images to relatively clear visual conventions. Clarity is itself invented: it is abduced from confusion.

Recall the abductive processes described in the famous ethnographic film about the Yanomamö, *The Ax Fight* (Asch and Chagnon 1975), in which the anthropologist first encourages the viewing student to experience bedlam and apparently random violence (all of this being iconic of what we are led to understand as the ethnographer's own original experience in the field), only to see snatched from tumultuous chaos the very ordered mechanics of a kinship diagram with appropriate accretions of demographic and historical data. We then re-view the chaos, and so are educated in its orderliness (as well as in the anthropologist's analytic skill).

It is perhaps ironic that an anthropologist often derided for his scientism should so exemplarily have displayed the very abductive process that scientism denies, and that lies at the heart of all the analyses presented here. The temptation of the heroic pose (Sontag 1970) can reveal a great deal of humanity in apparently mechanistic methods. When we discover these processes at work in medical practice, we should hardly be surprised at their occurrence in our own discipline; but perhaps it does take the disclosive force (see Crick 1976) of such comparisons to shock us into accepting what, we then tell ourselves in rueful self-justification (or professional intimacy), the scientists have apparently known all along.

The essays in this book thus have an epistemological force that their rather modest framing as being about the recovery of vision for anthropology might lead some readers to overlook. Because epistemology and ideology go hand-in-hand, the dampening of 'politics' as a theme may occlude the epistemological significance of the essays for some readers. To ask for a greater recognition of vision is thematic and methodological. To ask what the consequences of that shift will be for our own framing of anthropological knowledge goes much further. It is reflexive in a more specific and accessible sense than some of the more self-indulgent exercises that go by that name. These authors have largely chosen to focus on the practice of the new reflexivity, rather than on the political implications of the visual for a global critique. But this is a choice of emphasis rather than of substance. I have seen as my primary task the formulation of a complementary focus on some of the same concerns.

If the hindsight that we call 'abduction' offers insight into the 'enskilling' of vision, it would not take much of a second sight – abduction raised to the status of an 'uncanny' talent – to understand why the recovery of vision as a topic for anthropological investigation can relaunch, in new directions and modalities, the comparativism as well as the self-criticism that have always been the twin sides of the anthropological coin. To do so, however, we must also ask about the dangers of a deskilling of vision as well. Is the deskilling of our community of scholars what the rationalities of the twenty-first century hold in store? There are disquieting signs of such a trend, in which, then, the restless probing of anthropology will be seen as yet another impertinence deserving marginalisation. That reaction, with all the dangers it implies for what we conceive knowledge to be, would nevertheless only confirm the accuracy of our collective aim. As such, it might serve to open a deeply necessary debate, in which anthropology could once again be a voice to be heard – and a skilled vision to be seen – in the public sphere.

References

Abu-Lughod, L. 1990. 'The Romance of Resistance: Tracing Transformations of Power through Bedouin Women', *American Ethnologist* 17: 41–55.

Asch, T., and N.A. Chagnon. 1975. *The Ax Fight*. Film. Watertown, Mass.: Documentary Educational Resources.

Blum, J. 2000. 'Degradation without Deskilling: Twenty-Five Years in the San Francisco Shipyards', in *Global Ethnography: Forces, Connections, and Imaginations in a Postmodern World* ed. Michael Burawoy. Berkeley: University of California Press, 106–36.

Bourdieu, P. 1977. *Outline of a Theory of Practice*, trans. Richard Nice. Cambridge: Cambridge University Press.

de Certeau, M. 1984. *The Practice of Everyday Life*, trans. Steven F. Rendall. Berkeley: University of California Press.

Crick, M. 1976. *Explorations in Language and Meaning: Towards a Semantic Anthropology*. New York: John Wiley.

Douglas, M. 1966. *Purity and Danger: An Analysis of Concepts of Pollution and Taboo*. London: Routledge & Kegan Paul.

———. 1975. *Implicit Meanings: Essays in Anthropology*. London: Routledge & Kegan Paul.

———. 1986. *How Institutions Think*. Syracuse: Syracuse University Press.

Eco, U. 1976. *A Theory of Semiotics*. Bloomington: Indiana University Press.

Fabian, J. 1983. *Time and the Other: How Anthropology Makes Its Object*. New York: Columbia University Press.

Fernandez, J.W. 1974. 'The Mission of Metaphor in Expressive Culture', *Current Anthropology* 15: 119–45.

Gellner, E. 1983. *Nations and Nationalism*. Ithaca: Cornell University Press.

Goody, J. 1977. *The Domestication of the Savage Mind*. Cambridge: Cambridge University Press.

Herzfeld, M. 1987. *Anthropology through the Looking-Glass: Critical Ethnography in the Margins of Europe*. Cambridge: Cambridge University Press.

———. 2004. *The Body Impolitic: Artisans and Artifice in the Global Hierarchy of Value*. Chicago: University of Chicago Press.

———. 2005. *Cultural Intimacy: Social Poetics in the Nation-State*. New York: Routledge.

Hodgen, M.T. 1964. *Early Anthropology in the Sixteenth and Seventeenth Centuries*. Philadelphia: University of Pennsylvania Press.

Lévi-Strauss, C. 1983. *Le regard eloigné*. Paris: Plon.

Marcus, G.E. 1992. *Lives in Trust: The Fortunes of Dynastic Families in Late Twentieth-Century America*. With Peter Dobkin Hall. Boulder: Westview Press.

Needham, R. 1972. *Belief, Language, and Experience*. Oxford: Blackwell.

Rabinow, P. 1977. *Reflections on Fieldwork in Morocco*. Berkeley: University of California Press.

———. 1989. *French Modern: Norms and Forms of the Social Environment*. Cambridge, Mass.: MIT Press.

Raheja, G.G. 1996. 'Caste, Colonialism, and the Speech of the Colonized', *American Ethnologist* 23: 494–513.

Reed-Danahay, D. 1996. *Education and Identity in Rural France: The Politics of Schooling*. Cambridge: Cambridge University Press.
Scott, J.C. 1985. *Weapons of the Weak: Everyday Forms of Peasant Resistance*. New Haven: Yale University Press.
——. 1998. *Seeing Like a Stat: How Certain Schemes to Improve the Human Condition Have Failed*. New Haven: Yale University Press.
Sontag, S. 1970. 'The Anthropologist as Hero', in *Lévi-Strauss: The Anthropologist as Hero*, ed. E. Nelson Hayes. Cambridge, Mass.: MIT Press, 184–96.
Vernier, B. 1991. *La genèse sociale des sentiments: aînés et cadets dans l'île grecque de Karpathos*. Paris: Éditions de l'École des Hautes Études en Sciences Sociales.

Notes on Contributors

Daniela Bleichmar, Princeton Ph.D. in History of Science, is Assistant Professor in the Department of Art History and Spanish and Portuguese at the University of Southern California

Simon Cohn is Lecturer in Social Anthropology at Goldsmith College (University of London) and is currently engaged in ethnographic research on neuroscientific imaging technology.

Cristina Grasseni is Lecturer in Cultural Anthropology at the University of Bergamo (Italy), where she teaches at the Doctoral School in the Anthropology and Epistemology of Complexity (CE.R.CO.). Her monograph *Developing Vision, Developing Skill* is forthcoming with Berghahn Books.

Wendy Gunn coordinated the A.H.R.C.-funded project 'Learning Is Understanding in Practice: Exploring the Interrelations between Perception, Creativity and Skill' at the School of Fine Art, University of Dundee and the Anthropology Department, University of Aberdeen. She is Associate Professor of Design Anthropology at the Mads Clausen Institute, University of Southern Denmark.

Michael Herzfeld, Professor of Anthropology at Harvard University, has conducted research in Greece, Italy and Thailand, focusing predominantly on the politics of history and the inculcation of cultural and social values.

Andreas Roepstorff is Associate Professor of Social Anthropology and coordinates research at the Centre for Functionally Integrative Neuroscience at the University of Aarhus (Denmark).

Francesco Ronzon teaches Cultural Anthropology at the Academy of Fine Arts, Verona (Italy). He has conducted ethnographic fieldwork in Haiti, New York and in the gay community of Verona.

Barry Saunders is Assistant Professor of Social Medicine and Adjunct Assistant Professor of Anthropology and Religious Studies at University of North Carolina. His forthcoming monograph, *CT Suite: the Work of*

Diagnosis in the Age of Non-invasive Cutting, analyses the apprenticeship of the medical gaze in radiology.

David Turnbull has published extensively on the sociology and history of scientific knowledge, meant as a 'messy', situated social practice (*Masons, Tricksters and Cartographers*, 2000). He is currently an Honorary member of Deakin, Melbourne and Monash Universities, Australia.

Rane Willerslev is Lecturer in Visual Anthropology at the Granada Centre for Visual Anthropology, Manchester University. He has conducted fieldwork and made an ethnographic documentary amongst the Yukaghirs, a group of hunter-gatherers in Siberia.

Index

www.ingramcontent.com/pod-product-compliance
Lightning Source LLC
Chambersburg PA
CBHW072118020426
42334CB00018B/1644

9781845457037